'I think that the most important thing
a woman can have – next to talent,
of course – is her hairdresser.'
JOAN CRAWFORD

'I do maintain that if your hair is wrong,
your entire life is wrong.'
MORRISSEY

'I'm a big woman. I need big hair.'
ARETHA FRANKLIN

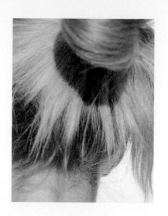

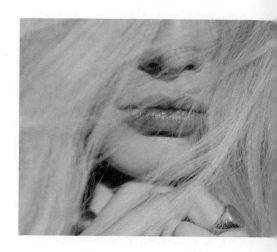

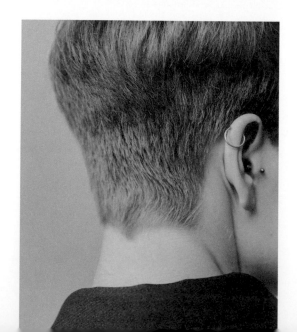

LUKE HERSHESON

GREAT HAIR DAYS & HOW TO HAVE THEM

EBURY
PRESS

FOREWORD BY VICTORIA BECKHAM

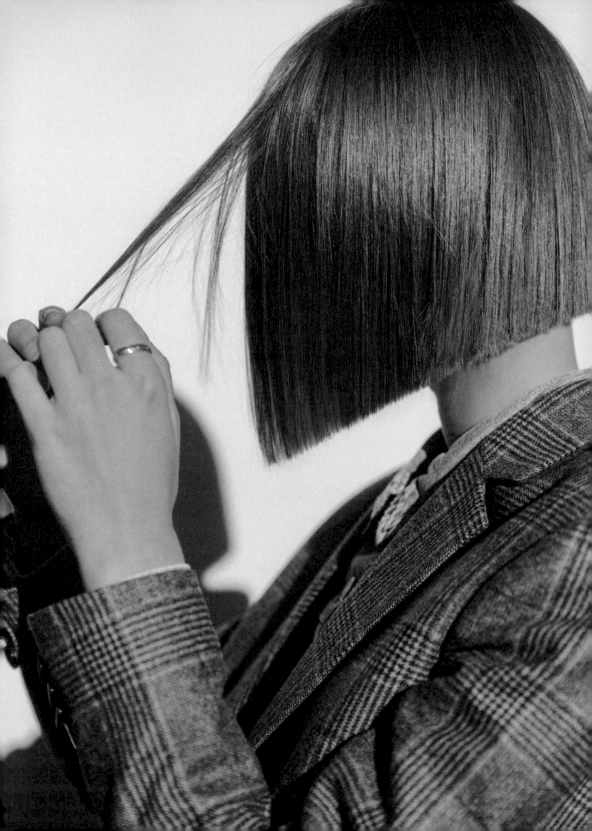

Luke is someone I trust implicitly with my hair – and that for me is key. He has a knowledge and experience so rich and varied that I feel comfortable listening to his suggestions, trying out new things and also importantly, just as happy to have what could be considered differences of opinion! And that's what's so refreshing. We have experimented, we have tonged and straightened, cut and lengthened – for editorial, for events, or just simply for me – and through each process I have learnt a little bit more about what I do and don't like for my hair.

Our hair is the starting point for feeling and looking good for all of us women. It's a fundamental part of our identity, our confidence, our look. Yet it can drive us to distraction. And here finally is our handbook to simplify and understand what we can do and how to achieve the best results – without (and excuse the pun) literally tearing our hair out.

I'm so excited that everyone can now share in Luke's expertise. This book brings together the answers to all our questions, provides invaluable advice for good and bad hair days and gives us all the help we need at our fingertips. Enjoy!

X VB

INTRODUCTION
BY
SALI
HUGHES

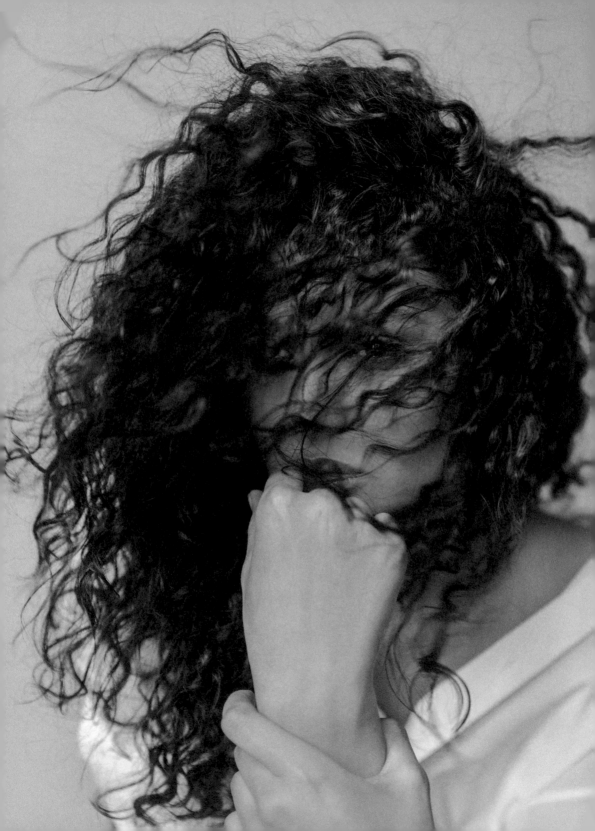

Just as there was life before the iPhone, retinol, gel manicures and Netflix, and will be afterwards, my life in hair can be divided into two distinct eras: B.H. and A.H. – Before Hershesons and After Hershesons. Though B.H. could just as well stand for bad hair.

From an early age, my passion for all things beauty was made easy by an almost instinctive understanding of skincare and make-up. But good hair – the third point of the triangle – didn't come anything like as naturally to me. From as far back as I can remember, my hair and I were in a dysfunctional relationship, swinging perpetually between embittered battle, when I'd grab crimpers, bendy rollers, clips or Carmens and attempt to force it into seemingly 'foolproof' looks from magazines (and invariably end up with achy arms, superficial skin burns and a sad, frizzy kink in my usual style), and the other extreme where I ignored my hair altogether and got on with my day while it sat there looking damp and piteous. As I entered adulthood, spent and defeated, this latter mode prevailed. Hair just wasn't my 'thing'. I couldn't do it, was blinded by science. I lacked the requisite coordination to master the two-armed dance between round brush and blow dryer, the patience for separating hair into uniform sections, the skill needed to create curls, the volume to keep any style in place beyond breakfast. So I simply opted out – leaving my hair to dry naturally in a lank, shapeless curtain while I attempted to pull focus with good brows and a bold lip.

It's entirely true to say that in almost every amateur photo that exists of me pre-2013, my hair – flat and forgotten, either ten years too old or too young for my face – looks nothing short of atrocious. The only time it ever looked decent was immediately after a haircut or professional blow dry and even as I pulled on my coat to leave the salon, I was already wondering how little social mileage I'd get from it before the whole thing reverted to its usual *meh*. A 'good' haircut was a one-day deal, a cruel snapshot of what I could have won, if only I weren't so utterly incapable of recreating the simplest of styles. I'd see others with braids, surfer-girl waves, up-dos and big, pouffy bedheads and wondered how on earth I missed the memo. If it needed anything more than a swish-through with straighteners (and let's face it, everything post-*Friends* and Cat Deeley rightly did), I counted myself out. For a very long time, despite my life being surrounded by the world's leading experts, I hated hair and the feeling was visibly mutual.

It's very odd to recall my life B.H., since – and please indulge my incredulous boasting here – I'm now really very bloody good at doing my own hair. I can make it photo-shoot ready in ten minutes flat. People on social media ask for tips on how to get it looking like that, even when I've just done it in the back of a cab. I can cheat a pro blow dry and breeze through three whole days before it starts to look grubby. Professional TV hairstylists have taken one cursory glance at my DIY do and ushered me on-set having decided to take no further action. I'm even told that women occasionally take my photo into the salon and ask for my hair. Me! The person with a terrible, fine, flyaway mop and sub-zero natural aptitude for styling it! How? The entirely honest answer begins and ends with one salon.

A little over five years ago, having spent over two decades dating, rebound-ing and cheating on all the big London salons, I finally discovered true love and monogamy at 45 Conduit Street. From the moment Luke Hersheson cut off my long locks, grabbing fistfuls of strands and hacking into them as though felling forestry, I finally began to understand my own hair. From that appointment forward, he and the team taught me that hair is really not that hard – and what's more, it actually looks a whole lot *better* when it's not. That doesn't mean I was on the right track when I combed it wet and left it to its own devices. It means that like that of a good cook, florist or cocktail waiter, Hershesons' approach is about taking three or four simple ingredients, and making something seem effortlessly beautiful.

What Luke, Adrian P., Jordan, Hadley, Grace, Sean and all the others have consistently taught me, is that my hair and I are on the same side. It's not about beating my thin, wispy, plentiful strands into submission or worse, into big, smooth, improbable arcs (as all the previous salons had done), it's about treating it to the right tools, giving it a little more movement with my drying technique, a bit more texture with a single styling product. It's about binning the brush and getting my hands in there, about having the confidence to be casual, to stay on just the right side of unruly, to make little changes to mix things up and stay current. And most of all, it's about getting a cut that doesn't need a round-the-clock hairdresser to keep it looking great.

I wondered why everyone wasn't doing their hair this way, why so many were wasting their time with complex, over-coiffed styles and looking way less cool than if they'd had an extra half-hour in bed. My boyfriend (hardly the observant type) kept asking me if I'd just got my hair done when I'd spent all day at the laptop. My girlfriends would tell me how good my hair looked when I'd barely spent more than two minutes getting it ready to go out. One by one, I sent my crew, despairing and depressed with their inability to keep a good barnet, into Hershesons. One by one out they came again, evangelical and fully capable of maintaining their newly cool hair at home. My friend Lauren Laverne began to call Hershesons 'The Happy Place' and we all understood, shuddering at the thought of it not being there, and of all the good hair days we'd needlessly missed. For the first time in our lives, we actually liked our hair and knew how to work it almost as well as the professionals.

And before you assume any of us is one of those Mayfair ladies who pop out for a daily blow dry, tiny yappy dog nestled in Hermès Birkin, let me relieve you of that idea. I get a blow dry only if I'm hosting an event, having my photo taken for a magazine, or am attending something posh. On almost any other occasion, the thought of getting up at stupid o'clock to get my hair washed in London is unappealing to say the least. I have neither the time nor the inclination – only a bursting diary, kids to get to school, words to write and meetings to attend. I want to roll out of bed, get ready fast, have hair that looks fabulous all day. My friends are the same and I expect you are too. Don't worry. The life-changing joy of the Hershesons method is that we don't have to be clients, live in London, be rich in either cash or time, and crucially, we don't have to be natural hairdressers. We just need to forget everything we thought we knew about hair, and learn to play by different rules. Hershesons rules. Believe me – you'll soon be ruined for all others.

Sali Hughes, 2018

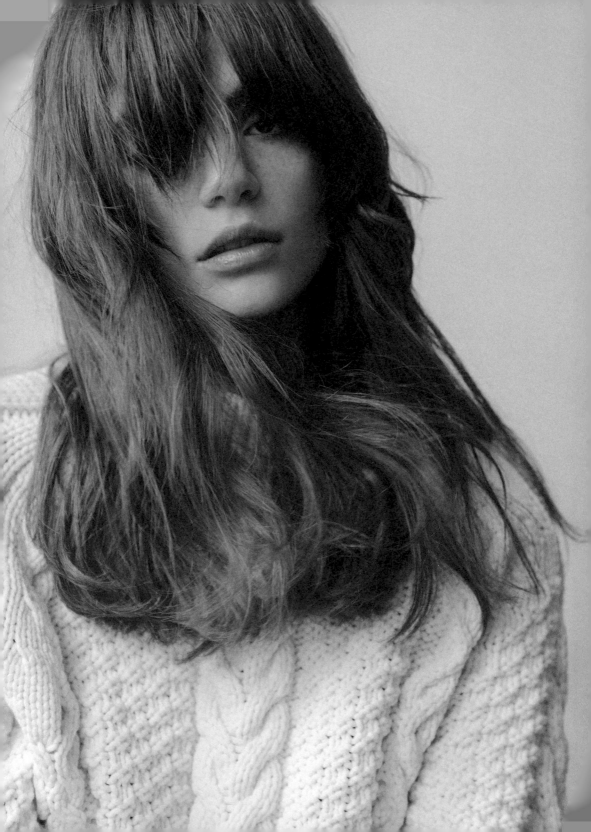

WHY HAIR?

'Hair is truly great when it is saying what you want it to say about you'

Any photographer, editor or fashion stylist will tell you that nine times out of ten it is the hair that is the real star of a shoot. Of course a great shoot is really a balance between the styling, the model, the make-up *and* the hair but from years of experience on-set I can tell you with confidence that if the hair is not right nothing else in the frame will work either. It is the linchpin upon which success rests. But hair doesn't lose its influence when it is no longer in front of the camera; in real life hair is just as – if not more – important. It's in real life that our hair really has a lot riding on it. It has a say in how we feel about ourselves, how others feel about us and how we express our true characters. And yet this hugely important aspect of it is also one of the least understood. Women who may have a strong sense of how they want their hair to look often feel intimidated or clueless about achieving it. The process and language of getting great hair can be foreign from the very first step into a salon, never mind when attempting to recreate it at home. I want you to know that I hear you. Our philosophy at Hershesons is not about trying hard, it's about getting it right. We know what you want, and in *Great Hair Days*, we'll tell you exactly how to get it.

I'm lucky that there has never been a time when I didn't know what I wanted to do with my life. I grew up in the salon watching my dad, acclaimed hairstylist Daniel Hersheson, cutting and styling and creating looks that were – in all honesty – completely ahead of the times. While other kids my age were probably playing video games, I was giving buzz cuts to my sister's Trolls with the clippers (sorry, Lauren), spending Saturdays with my dad at work sweeping, cleaning and shampooing, and styling the Girl's World my parents bought me to practise on.

My dad never actively pushed me in the direction of his profession – if anything he encouraged other things. But as far as I was concerned it was a foregone conclusion that I was going to follow in his footsteps. I toyed with photography and design for a time – I was even a milkman for about a week – but I just didn't want to do anything other than work with hair.

I know it's probably somewhat unusual to be so certain of your path at such a young age but hair has always inspired me. My dad opened his salon on Conduit Street in London when I was about twelve or thirteen; before that he had had other salons on Sloane Street and the King's Road, which in the eighties were the coolest places to be in London. I remember hanging out there at the weekends and seeing all these incredible people coming and going. There was an *Absolutely Fabulous* crowd at the Sloane Street salon who were very polished and after big blowouts, and glamorous Middle Eastern women with dramatically long flowing hair and chic English society stars. The King's Road salon was a hot place for punks so it really was the opposite end of the cultural spectrum. Between the two, I got quite an education in popular culture in all its variety. My dad's salons were *the* places to be and be seen. To me, that time in the salons summed up everything that was great about the eighties; it was really eclectic and there was a proper sense of freedom and fun, and at the heart of it all, great hair.

Generally underappreciated – certainly often neglected – hair is integral to your identity and pivotal to your self-esteem. How it looks, feels, smells and even moves tells a story; it speaks of your health, your age and your lifestyle as a whole. Not to oversell it, but evolutionarily speaking it is our most basic method of communication and a great hair day has the ability to completely transform mood and confidence. We would be unwise to underestimate it.

And let's not forget, there's a lot of money tied up in hair ($90 billion or thereabouts). People may underestimate the hair industry and mistakenly write it off as something frivolous but they couldn't be more wrong. Hair, like make-up, has the ability to defy the economy. When money is tight, people still find the cash to spend on their hair. Hair is the ultimate in comfort and its ability to shore up confidence is, frankly, priceless. That makes it pretty valuable in my book.

Hershesons has been a part of British hairdressing for decades and what we can tell you on the back of a lifetime of styling hair in the salon, on the catwalk and in front of the camera, is that hair is more often than not the star of the show. It's the glue that brings harmony between fashion and make-up and creates a 'look' – the entire thing can be turned on its head just by changing the hair. It's that powerful.

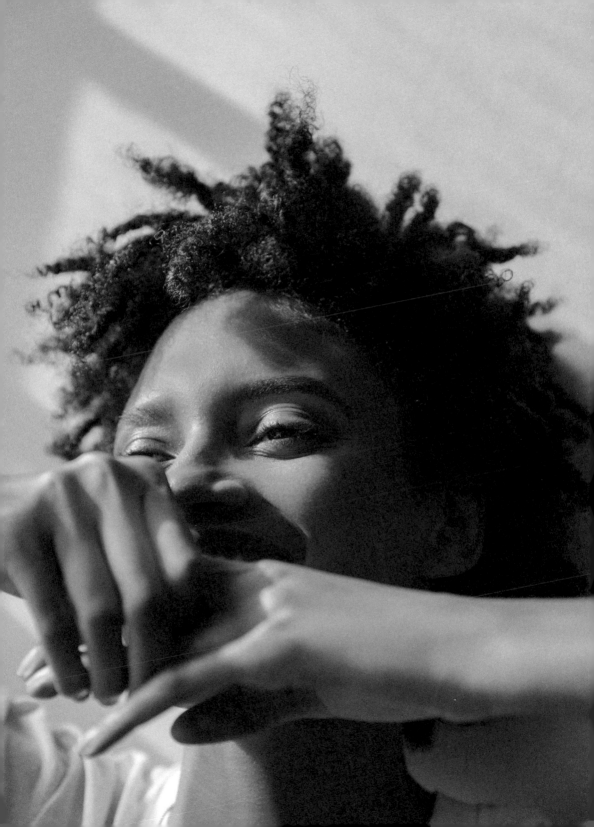

Throughout her life, a woman's relationship with her hair can, at times, be tumultuous; youth lends its vitality to hair with full and lustrous lengths, stress can result in hair loss, pregnancy can transform it entirely and hormonal changes later on in life can result in hair that's lacking in more ways than one. While it's undeniably a huge part of the feminine identity, hair is quite possibly the least understood aspect of women's (and yes, sometimes men's) appearance and they're often at a loss when it comes to understanding what it truly needs and how best to care for it – and that is, in part, down to conflicting messages from hairdressers and beauty editors and a near-constant assault of new products that claim to work miracles when, in fact, they do very little. No wonder people are so confused.

'Great hair' means something different to everyone; maybe it's freshly washed and glossy to the extreme, mid-length hair with just a touch of a wave, or maybe it's just-out-of-bed ruffled ends that hint of a night of mischief between the sheets. Whatever it means to you there's one thing for certain: great hair straddles a fine line between being too considered and being nonchalant, and there's a definite sense of empowerment and achievement that comes along with styling it yourself. But, even more than that, hair is only ever truly great when it is saying what you want it to say about *you*.

I believe that looking good and feeling good are inextricably linked and spending time and consideration on your hair is a worthwhile and rewarding exercise in self-care. If it takes an on-point haircut or a perfectly placed glossy ponytail worn with your signature red lipstick to make you feel equipped to meet a challenge head on – or take command of the room during an important meeting – then who is to say you're wrong? More importantly, who the hell has any right to label it wasteful vanity?

Your hair can have a much longer-lasting impact than the clothes you wear or the make-up you use. That all comes off at the end of the day, whereas your hair, that's something that is with you day in and day out and if you're unhappy with it, it's hard not to be unhappy in general. This doesn't just go for style-conscious women, I'm talking about all women. Whether you have created a specific style for yourself or you actually consider yourself to be unstylish and removed from fashion, if your hair is not doing what you want it to, or behaving in the way you want it to, it can get you down. Such is the impact our hair can have on our outlook.

You only have to speak to someone who has lost their hair to a medical condition or treatment to understand how it shapes character. Women who have lost their hair under these circumstances often say that it's this trauma that affected them the most on their road to recovery.

Understanding your hair is key to getting it to look and feel its best in a way that reflects who you are as a person, the lifestyle you lead and the people you identify with. And here's the great thing – it needn't be impossible to achieve yourself. Everyone, of all ages and all hair types, should have hair they love and with some expert tuition from us and a little bit of knowledge, *you* can become an expert in your own hair and ensure your look is telling the story you want it to.

I never want you to feel at a loss with your own hair again. I will share with you the tried-and-tested, suit-all-occasions styles that will see you through any event with confidence. We'll go right back to basics and look at your hair to really understand its characteristics and how to get the most from it. We'll cover everything, from what products you should be using and what you are likely wasting your money on, to how exactly you should be washing and styling your hair.

I chose to write this book because I want women to feel empowered when it comes to their hair; I want everyone to be able to walk into a salon with the confidence to tell their hairdresser or colourist exactly what they want, to be clear in their likes and dislikes so that their stylist can deliver, and know how to care for and style their hair at home so they look great and feel confident all the time. Great hair days are here to stay.

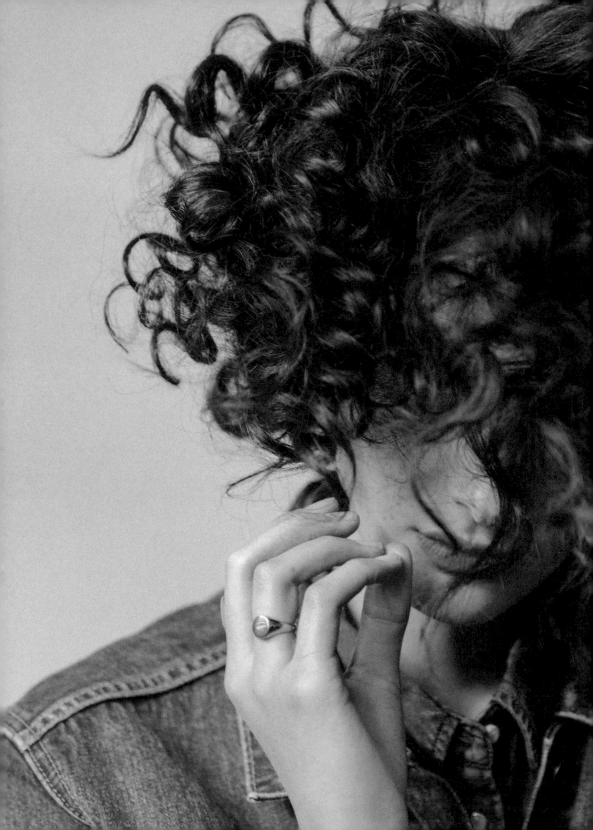

WHAT'S YOUR HAIR TYPE?

'Celebrate
what you have
been given and
enhance it'

You only have to look around you to see that hair comes in all shapes and sizes, and your own hair may look completely different from that of people in your social circle, or even people in your family. Maybe your hair is a mass of curls but your sister's is straight – it happens. But whether it's curly, straight, wavy or Afro, there are some things that all hair has in common and knowing more about the make-up of your hair will help you make better choices about it.

We each have around 100,000 hairs on our head and on average we lose 50 to 100 strands a day. Typically, blondes have finer hair and so they have more of them (around 140,000) while brunettes have somewhere in the region of 108,000 and redheads – who have the coarsest hair – have the least, only 90,000 or so. Generally speaking – and remembering there are always exceptions to the rules – Asian hair is the thickest and strongest of them all, measuring between 80 and 100 microns (a millionth of a metre), Caucasian hair measures between 50 and 80 microns and then African hair, which is the thinnest, only measures around 50 microns.

As a rule, each strand of hair grows for about six years before entering a three-month period of rest and dropping out. At any one time, 90 per cent of the hairs on our head are enjoying a growth phase while just 10 per cent are resting.

Hair looks pretty simple, doesn't it? Actually, it's anything but. Each strand is made up of the protein keratin (incidentally, this is the same stuff your nails are made up of) and if you were to look at one under a magnifying glass you would see that it's not too dissimilar from a rope. Albeit a tiny one. There is a protective outer layer called the cuticle, which is hard and creates a watertight seal to protect everything within, and then inside you'll find the cortex, which is what gives hair its strength and elasticity.

Virgin or unprocessed hair has a smooth cuticle, which looks something like intact roof tiles lying neatly over one another. This naturally makes hair look shiny and manageable and means it can withstand humidity.

Chemical treatments like colouring, perming and permanent straightening lift the cuticle 'tiles', which makes the hair vulnerable to damage. If you're naturally prone to frizz, that tendency will be exacerbated as moisture from your environment will be allowed past the cuticle where it will make your hair kink and curl.

The big question, the one that everyone asks, is how fast does hair grow? Well, this differs marginally between one person and another depending on how healthy you are, but on average you're looking at 5 inches of growth a year. If you're really healthy that measurement could be as high as 7 inches a year. I'll talk a bit later on about what you can do in terms of health and diet to get the most out of your hair.

HOW TO UNDERSTAND YOUR OWN HAIR

The first step to great hair is to know what you're working with. Dry, greasy or a little bit of both? Naturally frizzy or just over-processed? Damaged or naturally weak? Coarse and curly, or fine and poker straight? Nothing in a bottle will improve your hair until you really know exactly what you're dealing with. But there's one thing for sure: we're all guilty of massively misdiagnosing our hair. I've had clients who have 'warned' me that their hair is so curly, so coarse, so unruly, when the reality is something more along the lines of a wave or a few kinks. Most of us are long overdue an objective look at our hair, I think.

It's a good idea to understand your hair's texture, its porosity and elasticity, so you can judge what kind of intensive treatments it can benefit from and what, if any, chemical treatments you should avoid. If you don't understand your own hair how can you possibly know what it needs?

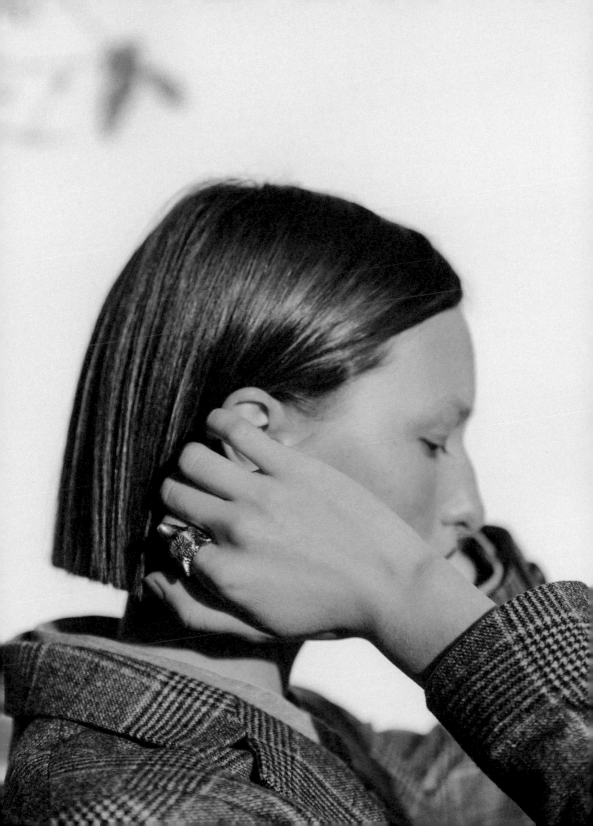

You should celebrate what you have been given and enhance it rather than feel that you have to change what nature gave you and conform to another hair type. On the whole, your hair texture shouldn't change much during your life – if you're curly you won't wake up one day and find that your hair has straightened itself in the night. That said, it is not unheard of for women to see textural changes such as more curls or a wirier feel after giving birth or once their hair has started to grow back following sudden loss.

STRAIGHT

There's a lot of beauty in straight hair; when it's in good shape it is glossy and luxurious but it has its downsides too. Straight hair ranges from baby-fine wisps that are almost impossible to curl (and when you do manage to add some shape the curl almost instantly drops out) to a super-thick mane of straight hair that might hide the odd wave or two underneath, takes a curl but frizzes up at the first sign of humidity. Straight hair can be thick, fine, frizzy or greasy and – thanks to its sleekness – it just so happens to be the shiniest of hair types. One-length straight hair can hang like a pair of curtains. Bizarrely, the more you chop into it the more life and guts you give it. If you cut it traditionally with very blunt lines, the hair will hang in a heavy way.

Straight hair can become greasy and limp pretty quickly and so it's important that it is washed frequently to prevent excess oils on the scalp from travelling down the hair shaft; dry shampoo should become your staple product as it will absorb oil and add a little volume and life. If you have fine straight hair you will find that the right cut is as much – if not more – important than the products you use.

Straight hair at a glance:
· Can be thick or fine
· Quickly becomes greasy and limp
· Frizzes at the drop of a hat
· Can be reluctant to hold a curl or wave
· Is often sleek and shiny

WAVY

If you have wavy hair, know you are likely the envy of women everywhere. But here's the thing: most women mistake their wavy hair for curls and frizz. Waves don't like to limit themselves and you're just as likely to have them whether your hair is baby fine or thick. Natural waves are the sweet spot between straight and curly hair, you just need to know how to make the most of them. Natural waves include everything from the occasional wave or kink to full and relaxed beachy goodness. If this is you, count yourself lucky, and just enhance what nature has given you. A great cut is essential if you want to make the most of your waves; some cleverly positioned layers and tapered ends will encourage more movement in your hair and make it easy as pie to style.

Wavy hair at a glance:
· Can be thick or fine
· Can include a handful of textures from a soft wave to more definitive kinks
· Is easier to style and manage when combined with layers
· Tends to be drier than straight hair

CURLY

For decades, curls have been on the receiving end of straightening treatments and flat irons, but thankfully curly women are finally learning to love them. This relatively new-found love of natural texture has resulted in more naturally curly models like Jasmine Sanders, Frederikke Sofie, Mica Arganaraz and Damaris Goddrie appearing on the catwalk and in advertising campaigns. In real life, women are rediscovering their natural curly texture too. Curls can lack uniformity – which I know some women find intolerable and a challenge when it comes to styling. You may have loose curls, which lack definition, cascading spirals, or tightly defined corkscrew curls, which frizz at any opportunity. Curly hair tends to be on the drier, more dehydrated side of things as the shape of the hair prevents oils travelling from the scalp to the ends and subsequently it may not feel as soft as straighter hair. Hydrating masks and products are essential.

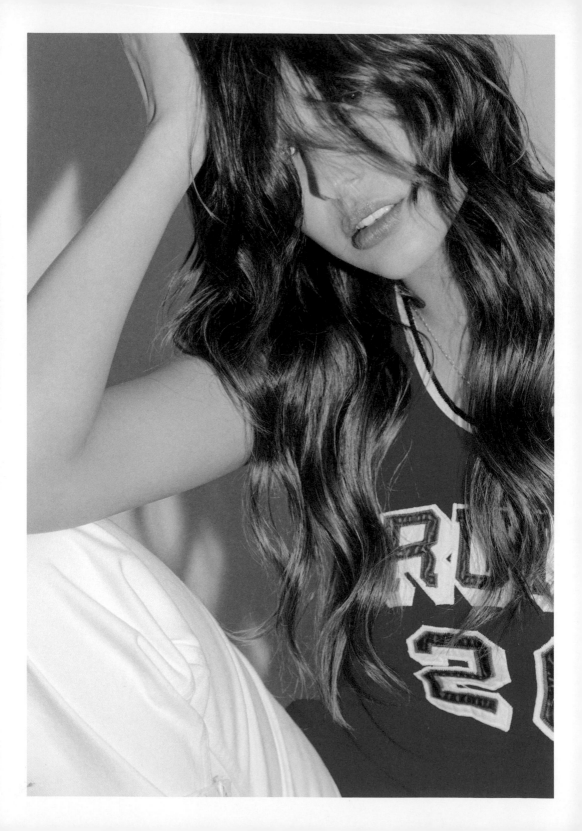

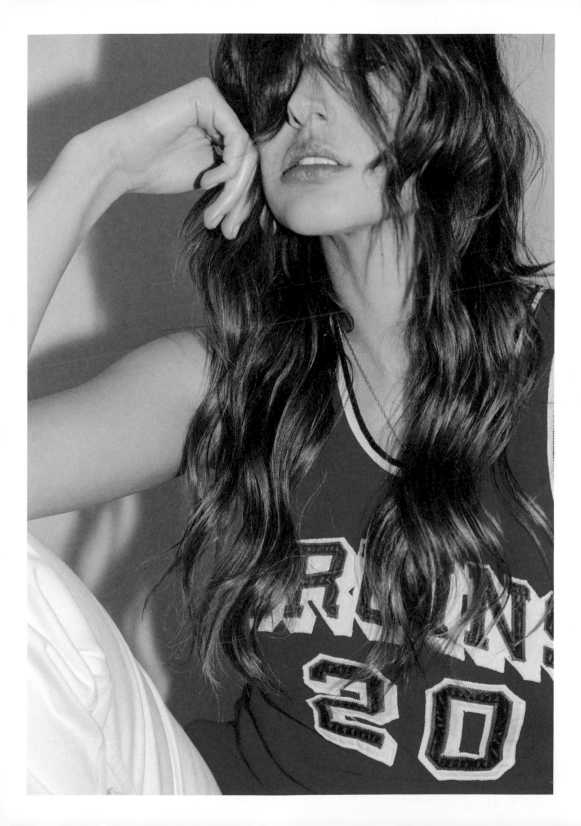

Curly hair at a glance:
· Curl shape can be irregular or uniform
· Hair is drier than straight and wavy hair
· Prone to frizz

CURLY COILS

Thanks to its many twists and turns, many women believe that coily hair is the trickiest to care for and style. I disagree, particularly when it comes to styling; I think that the lack of uniformity is actually a bonus and not a hindrance. It's what gives curly hair its character and makes it so cool. Think back on all those naff curly hair commercials in the nineties; what made those looks so terrible was that every single curl looked exactly the same. Absolute uniformity doesn't look natural. Moisture can be particularly troublesome to come by because oils from the scalp can have an extremely hard time travelling down strands, which can result in your coils looking and feeling dry and becoming brittle and prone to breakage. But with the right regime – and some discipline – this hair type can be all kinds of spectacular and it's refreshing to see so many women now embracing it. Coily hair includes everything from miniature curls and tiny ringlets, to a full head of glorious tight curls that lack any real curl pattern and can, unfortunately, be a complete nightmare to detangle. Diffusers can help bring some definition to hair with softer coils but if you have tight, dense curls then twisting your hair while still damp and allowing it to dry naturally is the best course of action.

Curly coils at a glance:
· Hair will be much drier than straight, wavy and curly hair types
· Texture can feel coarse
· Curl shapes range from tight coils to ringlets, irregular curl pattern likely
· Fragile and prone to breakage

MIXED TEXTURE

Then there is, of course, hair that is a complete mixed bag of textures. It's not uncommon to see hair in the salon that is relatively straight on top but with strong kinks underneath, or maybe an erratic and frizzy surface hiding much smoother hair underneath. Sound familiar? You are not alone.

POROSITY

Understanding how porous your hair is – that's to say, how easily your hair drinks in moisture – will help you to narrow down the products you should be using.

How do I know? Put a strand of your hair into a cup of water; if it sinks this means your hair is quick to take on liquids, but if it floats then your hair is non-porous and resistant to absorbing water.

But what does this mean? Well, if your hair is porous you likely have some damage that has lifted the hair's outer protective layer so it will suck up water-based products but is prone to more damage. Be sure to use heat protection before styling and maybe scale back on the chemical treatments until you have restored some strength and health to your hair. If your hair is non-porous then you can be pretty sure that your hair is in good nick and hasn't suffered too much damage. On the downside this also means that product is unlikely to penetrate very well and you may find yourself using more.

ELASTICITY

Testing your hair's elasticity is another way to quickly gauge damage and moisture levels.

How do I know? When wet, healthy hair should be able to stretch up to 50 per cent and still retract back into its original state, whereas dry, damaged hair will probably only stretch by say 20 per cent before snapping. Obviously don't test all your hair; one to four strands will do.

But what does this mean? If your hair isn't very elastic it's likely to be pretty parched and a little the worse for wear. If that's the case it's time to call in the big guns; rehydrating, rebuilding hair masks and serums are the order of the day.

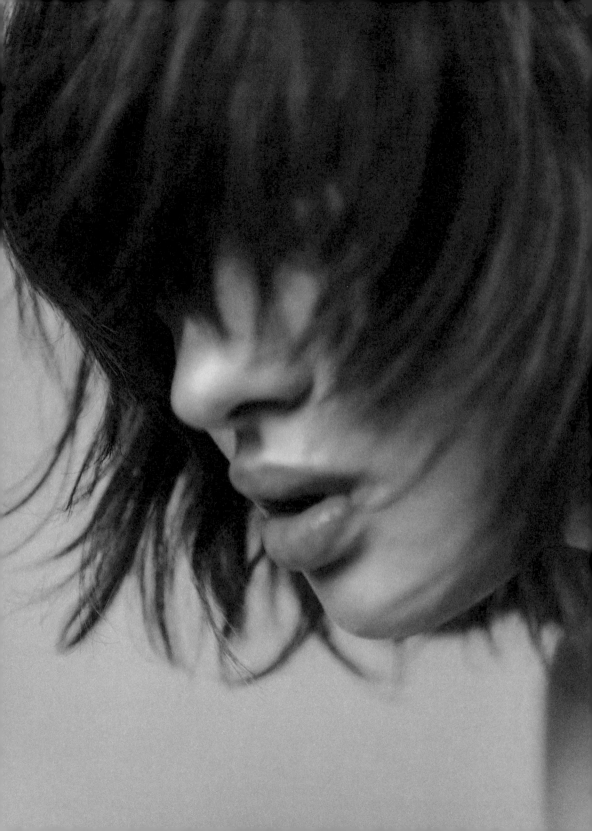

IT
ALL
STARTS
WITH
A
GOOD
HAIRCUT

'Behind every
great hairstyle is
a great cut'

If there is *one* thing that you take from this book I would hope it's this: the number one investment you can make in your appearance is in your hairdresser. I'm not saying this simply to big-up my profession; I'm saying it because without a great cut – even with all the product in the world at your fingertips – your hair will never do what you want it to. From the start, you're fighting an uphill battle. I have always been a firm believer that whether your hair is long, short, curly, straight, whatever, the cut is essential and if you get that stage right, everything else will fall into place. A cut doesn't have to be something distinctive, it doesn't have to be a sharp fringe or blunt ends, it could just be a little movement to encourage a wave or smooth buttery Sienna-style razored ends that kind of fall away to nothing. Ultimately it's a very simple formula; behind every great hairstyle is a great cut.

Classically, hairdressing has been about cutting the ends of hair – a trim or a bigger change to the length – and while that basic approach might have worked in the past when styles were more graphic, it certainly doesn't cut the mustard now. Before even picking up a pair of scissors, a hairdresser worth spending money on should be thinking about the distribution of hair from the roots right down to the tips; where they want density, where they need to add shape and, most importantly, what they need to do to deliver a look that you are happy to leave the salon with and will be able to style confidently and easily at home. This is why it's never a good idea to cut your own hair at home unless you are especially talented. There's a reason why hairdressers are trained to do what they do and that's because it takes skill to interpret your desires and create a style that looks as though it belongs.

Great Giselle-like waves in particular need a clever cut. You might think that slept-in and dishevelled waves are made all the better for not being cut. I can understand why you would think that; after all, it stands to reason that an undone, almost messy style like textured waves should, by its very nature, be low-maintenance and a cinch to achieve. Unfortunately, the opposite is true and often a lot of thought and consideration has to go into such a look. I suppose loose-textured waves are the hair equivalent of 'no make-up, make-up'; a whole lot of trickery and illusion goes into a style that suggests very little effort has been put in.

To enable the waves to fall just-so we cut in some invisible layers, which removes some of the weight from the hair and encourages movement, without affecting the length. Unlike more traditional layers that appear as a cascade of graduating lengths on top of the hair, invisible layers take a more stealth-like approach with a few hidden layers cut in from underneath. The result is hair that, to the eye, appears to be one length but is anything but.

If you were to try and achieve the same kind of beachy irregular wave – either with a tong or a soft perm – on hair that truly is all one length, you would actually end up with a very different effect. Adding a wave to one-length hair gives you something more solid, more clumpy, and a bit retro and graphic. That's great if that's what you set out to achieve but it's certainly not loose and relaxed, nor does it resemble fresh-from-the-surf beachy texture.

Perfect curls also demand a good cut and many women say that they don't fall in love with their curls until they discover the right one. Whether naturally occurring or permed into existence, a good cut is *always* behind a great head of curls. I think the reason why perms have been the subject of such scorn for the last couple of decades is because women still associate a perm with Charlene from *Neighbours* or the eighties Bubble Perm. They think perm and they think huge, round, poodle hair. But in reality that is entirely the fault of the cut, not the perm. If you leave length to the hair and add some layers around the front you can create something just amazing; the curls are tumbling, there's body where you want it, and overall the look is much fresher and simpler. Think Julia Roberts and Christy Turlington. I want nothing more than for people to stop thinking of a cut as something dramatic and definitive; it's not just about removing length, or cutting in a fringe – a good cut is so much more than that.

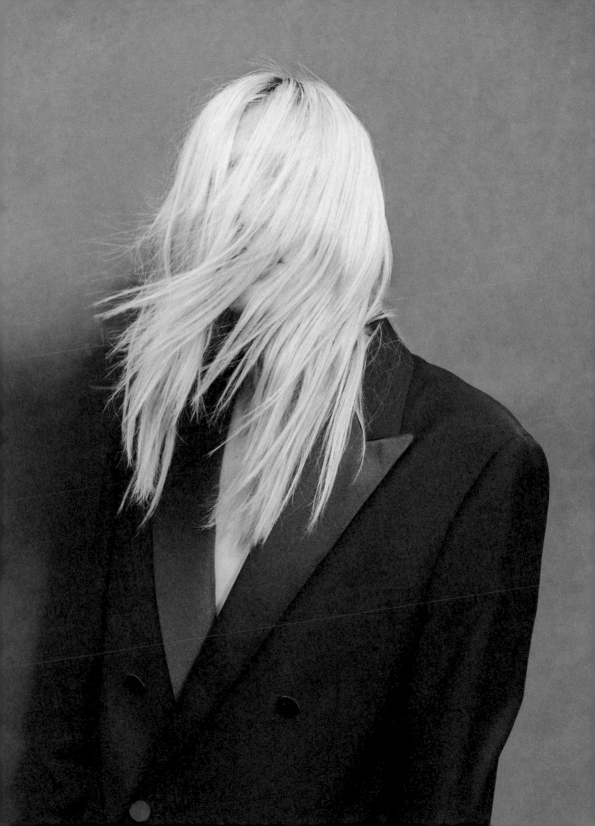

Unfortunately, plenty of women still leave their salon either frustrated or disappointed, or both, and I think this is down to not being challenged or nudged in the right direction. This is what separates the good hairdressers from the average; most hairdressers stand behind the chair, ask you what you want, nod their head politely and will make a decent attempt at creating that. In my book, that's just not enough. Of course, you may have a signature look that has been with you for years, or you may be happy to stay within your comfort zone, but I think what makes a *really* great hairdresser or colourist is someone who has an opinion, who can listen to what you want but also really look at you and maybe point you in a slightly different direction. Anyone can be taught to cut hair in a straight line, or cut in a few layers, but a great hairdresser should not just be someone who is technically good; they should be someone whose taste you respect, who has good style, and who can stand there and talk you through all of the possibilities open to you and make you feel excited and inspired. A great hairdresser should give you something you didn't even know you wanted – because they are an expert.

I still teach quite a lot and I tell every stylist I work with they must have an opinion. There's no right or wrong to this – an opinion is entirely subjective – and as the client, you of course always have the option to say no, but that stylist should be using their expertise and experience to help you decide what you want. I would hope that people come into our salons not just because they want a cut or a colour but because they want our input, our opinion, and maybe they want to try something slightly out of the ordinary for them.

I believe this is the reason why some women form lifelong relationships with their hairdressers. It's not unheard of for a client–hairdresser relationship to last longer than some friendships and even marriages. It's not just about picking up a pair of scissors and cutting someone's hair; as a hairdresser you are in an honoured position to accompany someone on their style journey and that requires a hell of a lot of trust. A hairstylist is a bit like a personal shopper or an interior designer; they are someone who understands your style intimately and what you like and dislike, but at the same time who presents something new and interesting that you may not have thought of on your own. Something that may feel bold and a little uncomfortable at first but which you ultimately love. That's the value in a good hairdresser.

Embracing change keeps your style fresh and interesting. You certainly shouldn't feel as though you must step outside your comfort zone every time you visit the salon, but it is nice to introduce a new or different element every nine months or so. This shouldn't necessarily be anything drastic or life-changing; maybe it's just a subtle tweak to your colour or adjusting where your parting lies. Sometimes it's not always about going from long to short either; small changes can be just as impactful as the big ones. It's funny that in my personal life I resolutely hate change – I like to visit the same restaurants and the same places time and time again (it's a bone of contention for my poor wife) – but in the salon I embrace it. My job revolves around constant change and without that element of newness it would become boring both for the women I work with and for me.

Don't just settle on a salon because it's local; locality might work for a simple blow dry but just because it is walking distance from your house doesn't mean that it's any good. The best way to find a great salon is to get recommendations – if your friends have brilliant cuts find out where they go, if you love a colleague's colour ask them who does it. From there on it's about finding the hairdresser or colourist on social media, checking out their work and communication, communication, communication.

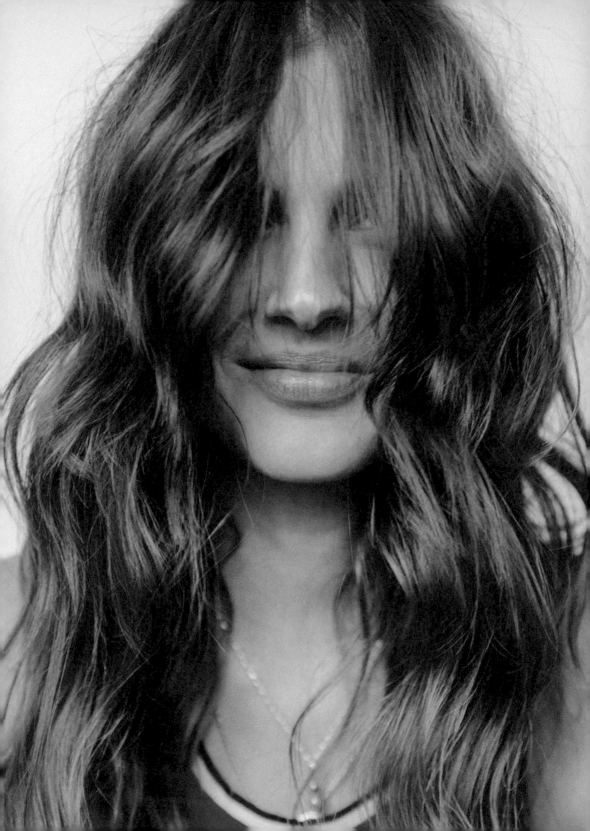

HOW TO FIND
THE RIGHT PERSON
FOR THE JOB

If you're thinking about trying a new hairdresser for the first time, do your research. You would research a painter/decorator before letting them loose on your house – so tell me why it should be any different for your hair. Remember, you will be living with the results of that salon appointment for some time. You need to know that your chosen hairdresser has a similar aesthetic to you and that they are technically capable of delivering what you want, and you need to see their previous work to make sure it's in line with the look you are after. I think it's completely unacceptable in this day and age for a hairstylist or colourist not to have a presence on social media. You should think of their Instagram account as their portfolio. Hairstylists should be posting pictures they're inspired by and looks they have created, so that their potential clients can see if they are on the same wavelength. If a hairdresser is not displaying their work in this way they are either not very proud of it or plain lazy.

Check out your salon's website too. At Hershesons we give each of our stylists and colourists a page on our site for them to talk about their style, skills, areas of expertise and what they're inspired by. I truly think this helps our clients decide on the right person for the job; it's also a great opportunity for our team to showcase themselves and their talents. Any good salon should be doing the same. Picking a hairdresser or colourist should not be pot-luck and based just on who's free at the time of your appointment.

IN THE SALON

I know that for many women an appointment at the salon can seem intimidating but it really needn't be. Remember, you're paying for that appointment, you are in the driving seat, so do not feel as though you can't speak up or that your opinion doesn't count. If you follow this advice you will rarely go wrong.

It's beyond useful when clients bring pictures into the salon. Of course, there is the odd occasion when the expectations are slightly unrealistic, but on the whole a picture is a valuable tool to communicate what you hope to achieve out of your appointment. Certain elements of hairdressing are subjective or open to interpretation. For example, one person's long is another person's short, one person's curly is another person's wavy, and one person's creamy beige blonde is actually another's yellow. Sometimes words are not enough but a picture cuts through all of that. Break the image down for your stylist. What is it that you like about the style? Is it the length, the texture, where the fringe falls, where the layers lie, the volume on top? Likewise, make sure you convey what you *don't* like. Be sure that you and your stylist are both singing from the same hymn sheet.

Beyond that, your stylist needs to be asking you all the right questions. They need to know how you tend to wear your hair, whether you blow-dry it, and if so whether you do it with a brush or with your fingers; how much time do you spend on styling your hair in the morning, do you like to straighten it? Everyone's answer is different. This kind of questioning should all be part of your consultation and is essential if your stylist is going to deliver a look that you're going to love and be able to style for yourself at home. There's no point cutting in a masterpiece that requires dexterous fingers and half an hour to style if your styling skills are limited and you have ten minutes to get ready in the morning.

Communication is a key part of the salon experience. I like to think that at Hershesons we never use jargon or hairdressy terms – that's just not the way our stylists are trained. We like to keep the language simple and descriptive so there is no confusion between us and the client, so when you come into the salon you're not left feeling completely bamboozled by terminology. I think the best hairdressers are the best communicators. Hair is not some weird artefact, and there's no reason whatsoever to make the process confusing.

An in-depth consultation before your hair is washed is more important than the cutting and styling itself and shouldn't need to take more than fifteen minutes or so. A good salon will provide this service for free. First of all, your stylist or colourist really needs to see you before you put your gown on so they can get an idea of the kinds of clothes you wear and your style. It's for this reason that we have changed things up in our salons. Instead of getting a robe on arrival and then being taken to your stylist or colourist, you'll meet the person doing your hair first and *then* they will get a gown for you. It's such a simple change but it really helps your stylist or colourist to get a feel for you as a person. If you are booking in with someone new, or if you are really stepping outside your comfort zone, I suggest having your consultation and then going home to think about the options given to you. Only then should you go back and get your hair done.

It's important to speak your mind and let your stylist know if you're unhappy. Some women are more comfortable than others when it comes to speaking up, and I know that sometimes it might feel easier to hold your tongue than to let someone know that you're dissatisfied with their work. But again it's important to remember that you are in the driving seat. I always think – and I could be wrong – that I can sense when someone is unhappy. As a hairdresser I think you should know, you should *feel* it via some sixth sense. This is another reason why the consultation element is so important and if a salon doesn't offer one for free, let me tell you, they are not worth your time or money.

There's no real standard that says how long your appointment should be or how often you should get your hair cut or coloured. A simple trim, for example, will take far less time than a completely new style. If your hair is damaged because of being heat styled every day you may suffer from more split ends and breakages, meaning you'll need to see your hairdresser more frequently. However, if you're pushed for time, remember to allow five to ten minutes within your appointment for your hair to be washed and conditioned at the backwash.

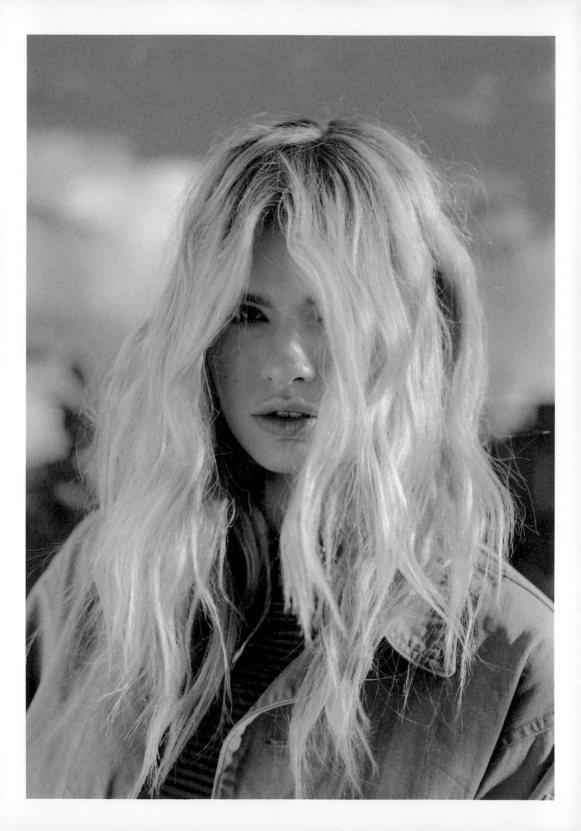

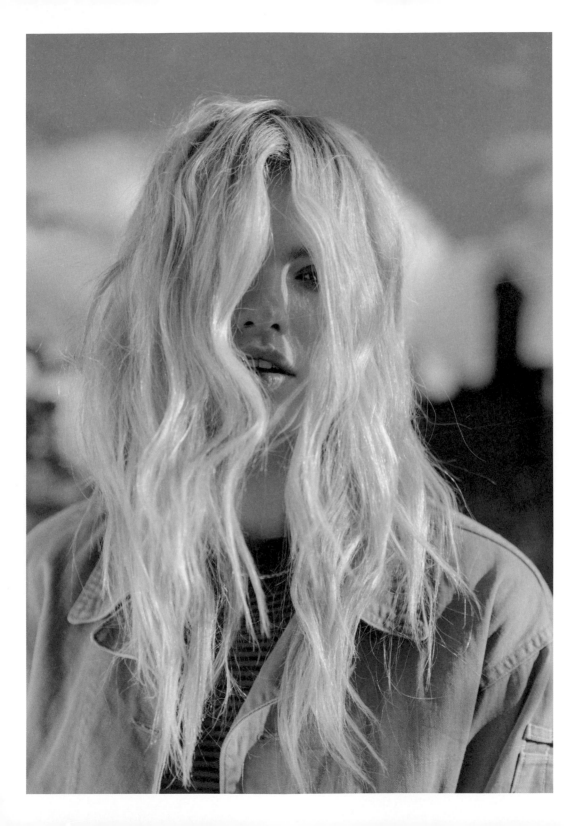

THE ENDS

Your hairstylist may talk about your ends a lot – I talk about them all the time – but this is because how your hair ends is just as important as your overall shape. Not every cut finishes in the same way and how your hair terminates can really influence the feel or aesthetic you're going for. Your stylist will take this into account when you're in the chair but here's what you can expect.

Smooth, buttery ends are the kind of finish you might see on someone like Sienna Miller. The ends are soft and ethereal and kind of melt away so you don't have any harsh lines. This is ideal for any kind of Parisian, relaxed, bohemian style.

Chunky ends are what you would see with a Bad Bob. They're choppy and almost look as though they have been hacked at with the kitchen scissors (in a good way, of course).

Blunt ends have a ruler-like precise finish and are the perfect partner to bold and graphic cuts.

THINGS A GOOD HAIRDRESSER SHOULD DO

Make you feel comfortable. Your hairdresser should make you feel at ease and confident to put your hair into their hands.

Ask questions. Your consultation time is an opportunity for your hairdresser to ask you questions like how long you have to style it in the morning, how often you like to wash it, how confident you are with a hairdryer, whether you like to wear your hair up or down and, most importantly, what you want to get out of your appointment. Do you want glossy and sleek hair, do you want something textured with lots of movement, or do you want something simple and low-maintenance? You both need to be on the same page.

Listen to you. If your stylist or colourist isn't really taking in what you want they are not going to deliver a style that you love. It's as simple as that.

WHAT TO DO IF . . .

If your stylist has made a mistake then you should be comfortable speaking to them about it and expecting them to put it right at no extra cost. But there's a difference between something being wrong and just not liking it. If your stylist has completely ignored your wishes, chopped off way more than you agreed or delivered a colour that is nothing like what you asked for, then the salon should absolutely do whatever it takes to rectify the issue. However, if, for example, you're just not sure of the shade of your colour, then you should pay for it, go home and live with it for a bit, and if you're still unhappy go back. A good salon worth your money will keep going until they get it right for you.

A WORD ON FRINGES

Fringes often need trimming more frequently than the rest of your hair, especially if you have opted for a grown-out eye-skimming fringe in the first place. Don't be tempted to trim yours at home unless you are very confident with a pair of scissors and know exactly what you are doing. Your salon will know that you will need to pop by in between your regular appointments for some fringe maintenance and most will do this for free. Do check with your salon though, as while this is the norm there will always be an exception.

AFRO CUTS

I firmly believe that cutting Afro hair is a specialism, so do not assume that every hairdresser does it well. At Hershesons we have a stylist called Amir Delijani who for more than the last two decades has dedicated himself to cutting coarse, curly and Afro-Caribbean hair types. He's extremely skilled and that's because honing this technique has been the focus of his career.

Cutting the curly and coily hair already mentioned in What's Your Hair Type? is a completely different discipline from cutting straight or wavy hair. The consultation needs to be more in-depth to spot signs of damaged or weakened hair; the cut can be more complicated as one head of hair can have multiple curl shapes; often the hair has to be treated before you can put a comb through it; and there is real skill in cutting hair that looks fairly simple when wet but becomes three-dimensional as it dries.

Your research is more important than ever when it comes to finding the right person to cut extremely curly and coily hair. Make sure you ask the salon for their dedicated stylist for Afro-Caribbean hair and look at examples of their work before you let them anywhere near you.

SALON ETIQUETTE

So, you've picked your stylist, made an appointment and you know what you want to do to your hair. Here's what to consider next.

Be on time. We understand that despite your best intentions there is always the possibility that you're going to be late. It's not the end of the world. If you're running late for your appointment be sure to call the salon as soon as you can to let them know. They won't cancel your appointment but it will give them a chance to shift things around a little. Your stylist or colourist probably has an entire day of appointments and just one person arriving late can make every following appointment run late also. Fifteen minutes is really the very latest you can arrive for your appointment and still expect to be seen or to receive the same dedicated time.

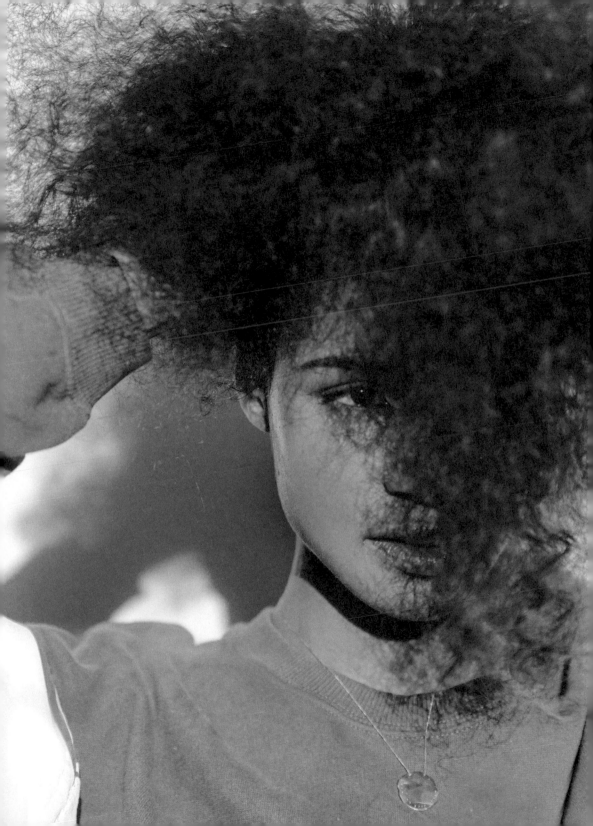

Communicate. Make sure you have had a thorough consultation with your stylist or colourist and that you both know what you're hoping to get out of the appointment. Talk about what you like and, importantly, what you don't like.

Bring pictures. Lots of pictures! Get descriptive and talk about everything you love in the image, whether it's the fringe, the length, the movement or the colour. A picture speaks a thousand words.

This is your time. It's no secret that hairdressers love a chinwag but if you're not feeling chatty you should never feel obliged to talk. This is your time to relax so do whatever you see fit (within reason, of course). Use this time to read a book, catch up on magazines or respond to texts or emails if that's what you want to do.

Be considerate. It's unlikely that it's ever a good idea to have a lengthy conversation on the phone with someone; it's distracting for your stylist and other clients.

Show your appreciation. If you're happy with your cut or colour then it's customary to tip your stylist 10 to 15 per cent. And don't forget the assistants who are washing your hair or bringing you a coffee. Tipping a couple of pounds shows that you're appreciative of their work too.

Don't disregard modelling. Granted, modelling for trainees is not for everyone but they are an affordable (or even sometimes free) way to try out a salon whose work you admire. It's a good idea when you really love what a salon does but you can't necessarily afford their prices. The appointment is certainly not as speedy as one with a fully trained stylist or colourist so you will need to exercise some patience. Remember, your trainee is properly supervised so there is minimal risk of walking out of there with hair you hate. But you must be realistic about what you are hoping to achieve out of the appointment as they won't have received the training they need to do absolutely everything and often things – such as a big colour change – need more than one appointment to perfect.

A word on pricing. I am often asked about the thinking behind different stylists being different prices and – to be truthful – there are a number of reasons why one stylist or colourist may be more expensive than someone else at the same salon. The price is usually a good indication of that person's experience and level of skill. For example, if the oldest stylist in the salon is priced as one of the lowest that should make you question whether they are doing really great work. On the flip side, if a relatively new up-and-comer is progressing through the pricing ranks pretty quickly then you can be fairly confident that they're pretty good. Price will also go up as the stylist or colourist gets busier; the more in demand they are the more valuable their time becomes. It's not uncommon for salons to give their stylists odd titles so it can be tricky to know who is more experienced in what. If you find the service menu confusing, don't be afraid to ask someone to explain it to you.

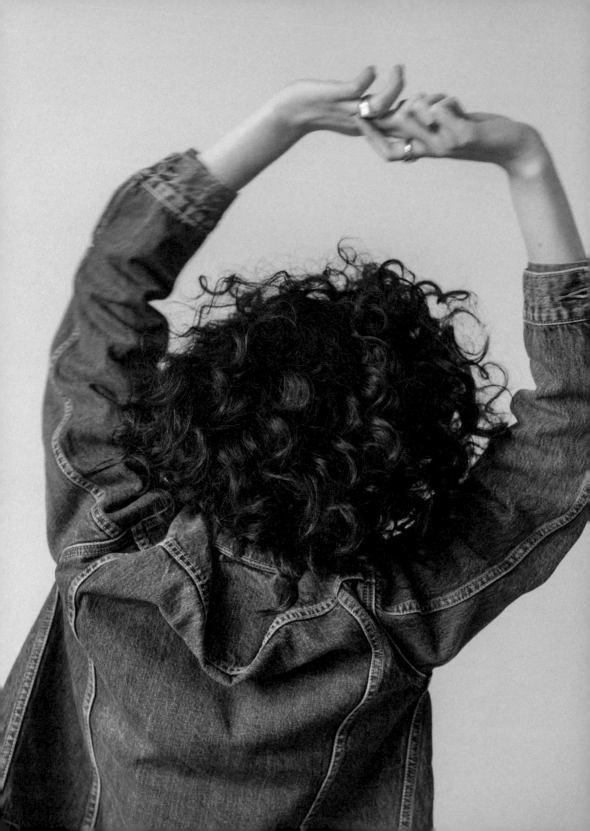

WHAT
YOU
NEED,
WHAT
YOU
DON'T

'Focus on quality rather than quantity and spend your money wisely'

It should go without saying that when it comes to your hair, your number one investment should be in a decent stylist and/or colourist. If you want great hair, I'm sorry to say, this first step is non-negotiable. But now you've got your amazing cut, how you style your hair and take care of it at home is still very important.

Unfortunately, the sheer number of styling products that amass on the average bathroom shelf is nothing short of mind-blowing. Women are thrown product after product and they're bamboozled with 'science' and clinical results (read the small print because many clinical studies are only ever carried out on a handful of women). Many products rely on good marketing rather than good results and here's the truth: most of the pastes, mousses, sprays and powders you're spending your hard-earned cash on are utter nonsense and will only end up in the graveyard that is your bathroom cupboard because they do not live up to their promises. The simple truth is that you don't need armfuls of products to create something as simple as a blow dry.

Every time a brand launches another 'must have' hairstyling product with a miracle claim or some pseudo-science attached to it, I hold my breath and hope for the best. I understand from the brand's point of view that newness is what their retail partners demand and the pressure that retailers put on brands to constantly bring out new and exciting products is relentless. This cycle of waste – waste of money, waste of time, waste of energy – is exhausting and more often than not ends with a customer disappointed that a product hasn't lived up to its claims. And really no hair brand needs fifty-odd products in its range because there are only a couple of products that actually improve how you style your hair at home.

Some hairdressers love to use loads of products, but that's just not my style. There is of course the allure of discovering something new, and I'm familiar with that traitorous internal voice that whispers, 'This is the one. This is *the* product that is going to transform my hair.' But it's all rubbish.

I'm sorry if that's not what you want to hear. Focus on quality rather than quantity and spend your money wisely; invest in a few tried-and-tested products that really do deliver noticeable results and make your life easier, and chuck the rest in the bin.

One area where we all benefit from a wide range of options is Care. As wonderful as some styling products are, they're mostly all fur coat and no knickers. That's to say that styling products really only work at a superficial level; while they can make your hair *look* great, they're probably doing very little for its overall condition.

When it comes to choosing the right care products for your hair (such as a weekly intensive mask) you really need to drill down to your most pressing concerns. Such as, do you have an irritated scalp, or is your hair particularly damaged? To make life more complicated, you most likely have more than one concern. Perhaps your hair is damaged *and* your scalp is irritated. It is for this reason – and quite rightly so – that there are a large number of care products on the shelves in-store.

Thankfully, many of the bigger brands are funnelling research money that once would have been spent on developing skincare into creating fantastic haircare products, which is why you might spot some more 'traditional' skincare terms and ingredients (such as 'anti-inflammatory' and antioxidants) in hair masks, serums and even shampoos and conditioners. To put it simply, haircare products are better now than they ever have been. This is what you need to know.

YOUR AT-HOME KIT

Before we get onto styling products, let's talk about the foundation of any hair routine: Care. Get this stage right and whatever styling products you use afterwards won't have to work as hard.

SHAMPOO AND CONDITIONER

Let's get the obvious stuff out of the way first, shall we? Whatever your hair type or concerns, a good shampoo and conditioner are essential. But not everyone necessarily benefits from using a traditional shampoo and may prefer to use the 'pre-poo' method of cleansing with an oil – I'll go into detail about this in Your Hair Routine.

At their most basic, your shampoo and conditioner serve just two purposes: to clean and to condition and/or hydrate your hair. The process of shampooing – coupled with the mechanical action of rubbing – lightly lifts each hair's cuticle so that it can remove dirt and excess oils. It is the duty of your conditioner to then swoop in, smooth the cuticle and restore lost moisture.

If your hair is perfectly ordinary – not chemically treated, not greasy, not dry, you don't have an itchy scalp, nor are you prone to frizz – then you *may* not need anything more than a shampoo and conditioner that effectively does just those two things.

If, however, you have any kind of hair concern – or your hair has had a chemical treatment such as a perm or even a colour – then you should be looking to address your specific needs with your shampoo and conditioner. As an example, some particular sulphates found in shampoos can be pretty harsh on the scalp and so they're not ideal for anyone with a skin sensitivity.

I am asked all the time whether it is worth splashing out on an expensive shampoo and conditioner or whether a bargain-basement duo will do the job just as well. I know you would love for me to say that this is an area within your haircare regime where you can get away with scrimping, but I would be lying.

Super-cheap brands tend to only work superficially. For example, many are packed with cheap silicones, which latch onto hair strands and make them appear glossy. The result is hair that may look great in the short term but without any long-term benefits whatsoever. Broadly speaking, more expensive brands (I'm thinking along the lines of Kérastase where a shampoo can set you back around £19) contain sophisticated ingredients, they spend more money in their labs creating really efficacious products, and their formulations are steeped in science. More expensive products also tend to contain finer fragrances, which may seem trivial but we all know how important it is for our hair to smell incredible. Essentially, premium haircare brands are called 'premium' for a reason.

My best advice is to spend as well as possible within your budget and research the range and the ingredients used before parting with your money. As mentioned, Kérastase have some exceptional shampoos and conditioners that address hair concerns such as lack of volume, damage, excess oil and thinning. I also wouldn't hesitate to recommend the botanical brands Phyto and Philip B.

John Frieda is a fantastic go-to brand for shampoos and conditioners specifically tailored for coloured hair. They really are streets ahead of other brands when it comes to enhancing and tweaking your colour at home. Look out for Brilliant Brunette, Sheer Blonde and Radiant Red ranges that brighten and intensify your bottled colour. Sheer Blonde Go Blonder In-Shower Lightening Treatment is particularly great; you apply it all over wet hair (in the shower), especially the roots, allow it five minutes to work its magic and then rinse out. The formula gently lightens your hair without turning the colour brassy.

Christophe Robin is another brand that really focuses on maintaining and enhancing bottled colour. The Shade Variations cater for redheads, brunettes and a couple of shades of blonde, and again just need a few minutes on your hair to enrich your shade.

Washing your hair is, sometimes, not as simple as it sounds but Your Hair Routine will break the basics down for you.

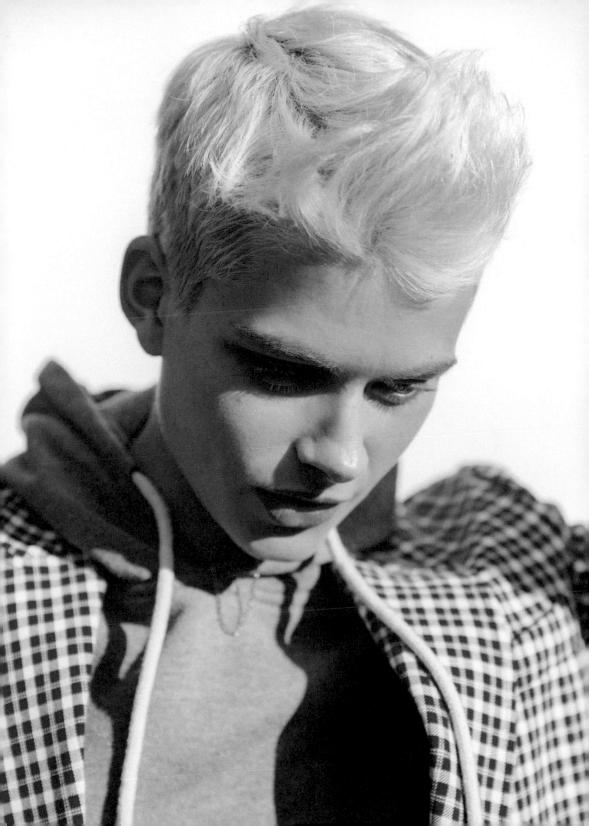

READING THE LABEL

Have a look at the ingredients list on the shampoo and conditioner in your bathroom right now. Do you recognise any of them? The ingredients are listed in order of concentration – water (or aqua) is usually the first on the list and perfume usually occupies the last spot. Here are the ingredients you need to know about.

Sulphates (often shown as sodium laureth sulfate, ammonium lauryl sulfate, sodium trideceth sulfate and cocamidopropyl betaine) are the main cleansing ingredients in shampoo and they're what creates a lather. If you have a sensitive scalp you may find some sulphates irritating – a trichologist (hair doctor) should be able to narrow it down for you, or alternatively you could try a sulphate-free brand such as Pureology. Body Shop Rainforest Shine Shampoo has also been formulated without any sulphates.

Silicones or siloxanes seal the hair's cuticle and make it shine. A lot of bad things have been said about them over the years, primarily because they can't be rinsed away and need to be removed with shampoos, so they can build up on the hair over time. This isn't necessarily a bad thing and you may have no problems at all with silicones, but they can feel heavy on very fine hair.

Sodium chloride is essentially salt, which sounds like an odd thing to put in a shampoo but it does serve a purpose. Sodium chloride roughs the cuticle up a little and so can make fine, flat hair look fuller. If your hair is very coarse you may not want to use a shampoo containing it.

Fatty alcohols often appear on conditioner labels as cetyl alcohol, stearyl alcohol or cetearyl alcohol. Despite being alcohols, they actually moisturise your hair. Fatty alcohols are great for almost all hair types, though if you have a sensitive scalp they may not agree with you.

Parabens are a group of chemicals that have been used for decades to prevent harmful bacteria from forming and preserve the shelf life of your products. They are a controversial ingredient that has received negative press (much of it inaccurate) over the years. Despite being demonised, parabens are deemed safe to use in small quantities in beauty products.

Salicylic acid is a beta hydroxyl acid (or BHA) and it's used a lot in skincare products to keep pores clear of bacteria and to treat acne. It works just as well on the scalp and that's why you'll find it in a lot of shampoos; if you have a flaky, irritated scalp then look for shampoos containing this clever ingredient.

Detanglers are used in conditioners for obvious reasons. The most common ones are cetrimonium chloride and cetrimonium methosulfate. Brilliant for coarse and curly hair.

Proteins are used in conditioners and masks to give the hair strength. Look for wheat protein and soy amino acids. Excellent for most hair types including damaged, over-processed and regularly heat-styled hair.

BEST IN SHOW
This is by no means a definitive list but if you're looking for a great shampoo and conditioner for your hair type, here is a good place to start. Remember, there is no rule that says you have to use shampoo and conditioner from the same range; if you have multiple hair concerns, address them with a different shampoo and conditioner.

Best for an itchy or sensitive scalp: Philip Kingsley Flaky/Itchy Scalp Shampoo contains gentle non-irritating cleansers and wards against the bacteria responsible for uncomfortable scalps. Incidentally, this formula was first created for Sir Laurence Olivier.

Best for Afro hair: Whether you like to use a traditional shampoo and conditioner or prefer a co-wash product (more on this in a bit) you really can't go wrong with the Vernon François range. The Co-wash Shampoo and Curl Command Shampoo and Conditioner are brilliant.

Best for greasy hair: Kérastase Bain Divalent is a shampoo that has been formulated to gently cleanse the scalp and regulate the excess sebum responsible for making your hair greasy. Crucially, the formula is silicone free.

Best for smoothing frizz and flyaways: John Frieda Frizz Ease Forever Smooth Shampoo and Conditioner are line extensions to their cult Frizz Ease serum. They do an admirable job of taming fluff and flyaways before you even begin the styling process.

Best for boosting thinning hair: Nioxin 3 Part System No.2 is a kit that includes shampoo, conditioner and a targeted hair treatment which you apply directly to your scalp. The packaging looks a little medicinal but the products themselves are brilliant. They create the right scalp and follicle condition for healthy hair growth.

Best for damaged hair: Phyto Phytokératine Extrême Shampoo is ideal for dyed, highlighted, heat-styled and over-processed hair.

Best for dandruff: Head & Shoulders Classic Clean Shampoo and Conditioner may not sound new or revolutionary but if something ain't broke, why fix it? Head & Shoulders famously contains zinc pyrithione, which eases flakes and that damnable itch. What it lacks in #shelfie status it more than makes up for in flake-clearing expertise.

Best for creating volume: Kérastase Bain Volumifique and Gelée Volumifique add volume and the illusion of density while still leaving the hair feeling soft and touchable rather than chock-full of product.

Best for coloured hair: John Frieda really excels at taking care of coloured hair whilst also preserving and enhancing colour. The Brilliant Brunette, Sheer Blonde and Radiant Red ranges are equally brilliant.

Best for dry/dehydrated hair: While some shampoos can leave dry hair feeling even drier, Philip B African Shea Butter Gentle & Conditioning Shampoo puts the moisture back in.

HEAT PROTECTION

Before you apply any kind of heat to your hair in the form of a tong, straightener or hairdryer, you should always use a product that will protect your fragile strands from the high temperatures first. Damage from heat styling makes hair look completely frazzled; it depletes moisture and erodes the outer cuticle layers making hair weak, brittle and a nightmare to style.

Your styling tool can exceed 200 degrees, which is a lot for your hair to contend with. Most heat protectors – whether in an oil or spray format – protect the hair from temperatures as extreme as 450 degrees and should be applied from your roots to ends – on wet or dry hair – before you reach for the heat. L'Oréal Professionnel Tecni.Art Constructor is a favourite of mine; it's a great heat protector but it also lightly texturises and gives a little hold. Philip Kingsley Daily Damage Defence, Oribe Foundation Mist and Living Proof Blowout are brilliant too.

SUN PROTECTION

I like to think that we're all pretty savvy when it comes to protecting our skin from the sun. We know that ultraviolet A (UVA) and ultraviolet B (UVB) rays damage skin in both the short and long term with burning being the most pressing concern and lines, wrinkles, sun spots and skin cancers affecting our skin long after exposure. Our skin habits now are completely unrecognisable from what they were just ten years ago and I'm willing to wager that next to no one lies out in the sun any more without adequate protection. But, while our skin is protected, our hair and scalp are mostly left to fend for themselves. UVA and UVB are just as damaging to our hair and scalp; various studies show that these rays weaken the structure of the hair shaft and deplete essential proteins (especially keratin). Not to mention that sun exposure literally bleaches the colour from your hair and your scalp is just as likely – if not more likely – to develop worrying melanomas as it feels the full brunt of the sun. From a styling point of view, UV damage leads to dry, brittle, breakage-prone hair – all the stuff no one wants.

Hopefully I've scared you enough into using sun protection on your hair and scalp. I do hope so. It's very simple: when in the sun treat your hair the same way that you would your skin. Use products containing UV filters plus protective ingredients such as oils and waxes and when appropriate wear a hat. Kérastase, Philip Kingsley, L'Oréal Professionnel, Davines and Phyto all have great leave-in products designed to protect your hair, and aftercare products that have been formulated to repair damage and mop up free radicals – the atoms that cause hair to prematurely age, becoming thinner, drier and more wiry. I love Phyto Plage Protective Sun Oil, a brilliant leave-in product that you can keep applying throughout the day as it doesn't turn oily and leaves hair feeling soft and silky.

Whatever you decide to use, the premise is the same: apply it from roots to ends – and over your parting – on dry or wet hair before going into the sun and remember to reapply after swimming.

A MASK

A weekly hair mask is by no means an essential but if you have a specific hair concern – such as damage or really dry hair – then treating it with an intensive mask can only do good things, plus chilling out with a hair mask on is good for the soul. Choose one that addresses your hair concern; if it's damage you're worried about – such as splits and breakages – look for a mask containing proteins (specifically keratin) like Phyto Phytokeratine Extreme Exceptional Mask; if you're trying to hang on to your bottled colour for longer, opt for a mask that deposits a touch of pigment to refresh your shade.

John Frieda have a brilliant range of intensive treatments that sharpen blondes and intensify brunette and red shades. Most brands – including Kérastase, Oribe, Leonor Greyl, Phyto, L'Oréal Professionnel and Philip B – cater for hair that needs an injection of moisture, shine, frizz management or colour protection. As a rule, anything listed on the ingredients label as a 'butter' will hydrate, add shine and detangle, and elastins and proteins such as wheat protein deliver strength – usually any kind of plant or fruit extract will be an antioxidant, which means it will protect your hair from UV and damage caused by pollution.

Get the most out of your weekly masking sessions by wearing a shower cap while allowing your mask to work its magic; the heat produced under

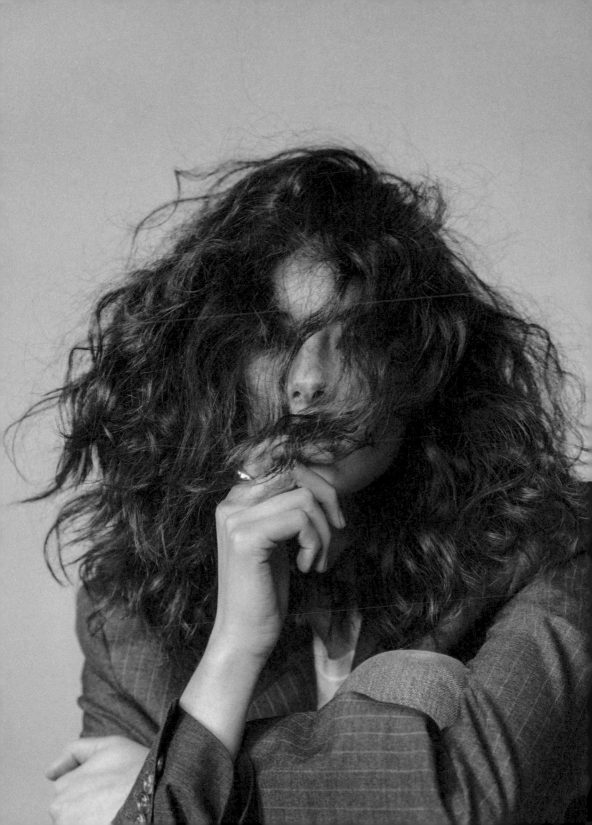

the cap will help it penetrate. If you're familiar with cocktailing your skincare products, apply the same philosophy to your mask; maybe apply a scalp mask with cooling and antibacterial benefits over your scalp and root area to ease inflammation, and mix coconut oil in with your hair mask to ramp up its softening properties before applying it to the rest of your hair. Use the directions on the pack as a kick-off point and bespoke the rest.

If your hair is particularly fine you might want to avoid using very thick and occlusive masks in a traditional manner as they may weigh down your fine strands. Instead, use these masks as a pre-shampoo treatment instead so that you get the rebuilding and strengthening benefits without the weight. Otherwise, all hair types can benefit from extra hydration and five to ten minutes with a mask.

TONICS

Hair and scalp serums are relatively new to the game but they're a brilliant way to introduce concentrated ingredients into your haircare regime. Just like a skin serum, a hair or scalp serum contains potent active ingredients in smaller molecules than you'll find in regular products; this enables the serum to penetrate further into the scalp and hair follicles to where it can really have an impact. A serum is not essential but it can make all the difference to the condition of your hair, especially if you're thinning. Depending on the formula, you usually section out your hair so that you can apply the serum evenly over your scalp. Rubbing it in with the tips of your fingers will help the product to absorb even better. Remember, healthy hair and a healthy scalp go hand in hand.

WHAT TO LOOK OUT FOR IN YOUR TONIC

These ingredients do appear from time to time in shampoos and conditioners but in order to do their thing they're needed in high dosages which is why they are perfect in a serum or tonic. If you're very diligent you *could* use a serum or tonic indefinitely as part of your haircare routine, or just use it for three or four months as an intensive course when your hair needs an extra boost. Depending on your main concerns, here is what you should be in the market for:

Thinning: Stemoxydine is a L'Oréal ingredient that creates the right environment within the scalp for new hair growth. You can find it in a bunch of L'Oréal brands including Kérastase Densifique, L'Oréal Professionnel Serioxyl and Redken Cerafill ranges. The industry gold standard, however, is minoxidil, which can be found in Regaine. You need to exercise some patience whenever you're using a product designed to up the number of hairs on your head because the results – while promising – usually take their sweet time (anything from three to four months) to put in an appearance.

Irritated scalp: Look for scalp serums, tonics or toners that contain cooling ingredients like camphor and anti-itch ingredients such as benzalkonium chloride. You'll find both of them in Philip Kingsley Flaky/Itchy Scalp Toner.

Damaged hair: Hair derives its strength from protein, but chemical treatments, heat styling and just day-to-day living deplete it. Serums containing small protein molecules will put your hair on the path to recovery. Keep an eye out in particular for serums containing the protein keratin as it's the most valuable to your hair.

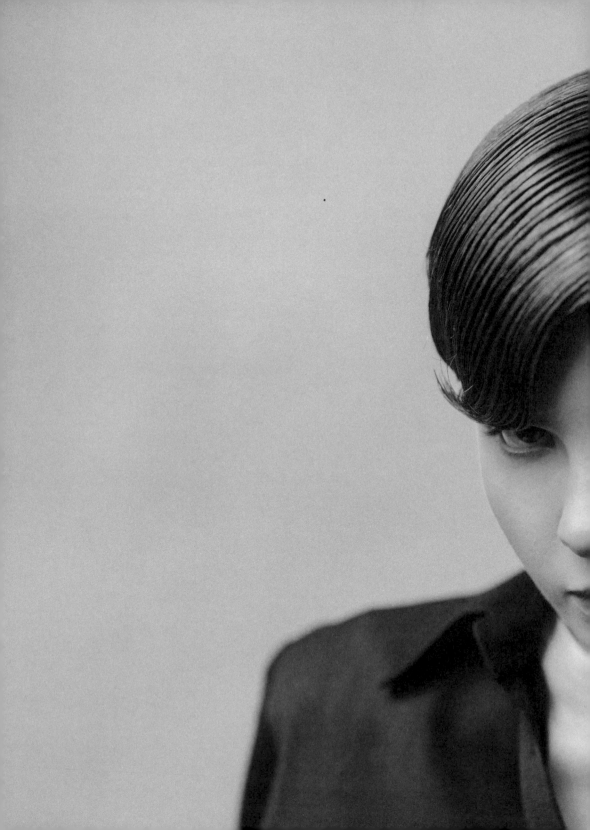

STYLING
ESSENTIALS

'When it comes
to what you do
need the list is
a short one'

Ordinarily you shouldn't be using more than two styling products in your hair at any one time. Whatever your hair type – or style that you're hoping to achieve – you really only need one wet-styling product and one dry-styling or finishing product. I have a problem with the sheer enormity of styling products out there; there's way too much on the shelves in-store and you just don't need most of it. When it comes to what you *do* need the list is a short one and – with the exception of hair oil, which really does its best work with curly and coily hair – everything is suitable for all hair types.

L'ORÉAL ELNETT

Once, when I was much younger and new to the industry, I worked with a very famous photographer on a shoot; he's the kind of photographer who really knows hair – he's obsessed by it. He caught me on-set with a random can of hairspray that wasn't Elnett and he took it from me and threw it across the room. You might think this was somewhat of an over-reaction but he was absolutely right to do what he did; after all, it is the photographer who really scrutinizes an image. He told me I should go through a can of Elnett a day, and again, he was right. I now use *at least* a can a day when I'm working on-set.

Hairspray is an overworked and often underappreciated product but we would be lost without it. It adds hold (whether your hair is up or down), it creates a lived-in texture, it sets a wave or curl in hair that would otherwise be pretty straight – it's nothing short of a miracle worker and I couldn't do my job without it.

And here's the truth: L'Oréal Elnett is the best hairspray ever created – for every single hair type – and even as someone who develops products I would honestly never consider making another hairspray unless I knew I could do it better. It doesn't make the hair wet, sticky or heavy, it can be brushed out easily and the more you put in the better the hair looks. It

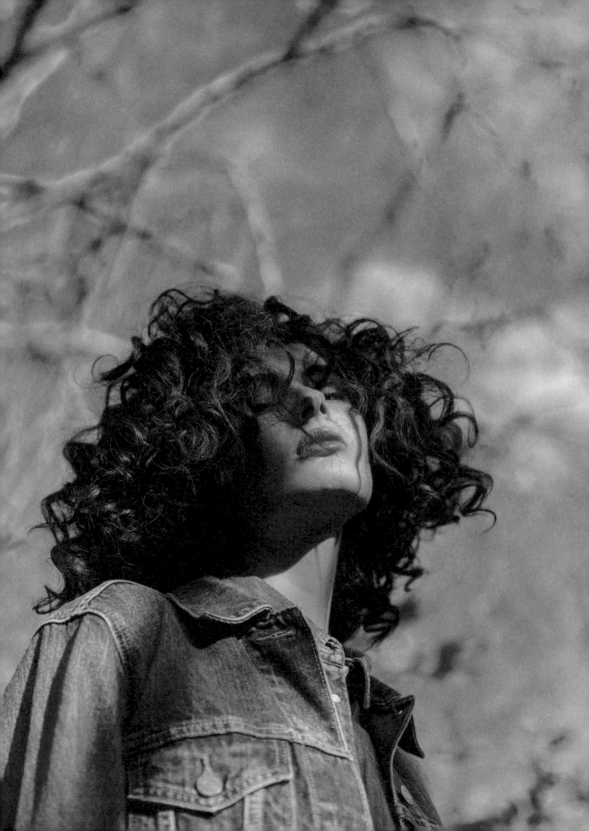

adds some oomph to freshly washed hair and makes it so much easier to style. Elnett can be used in different ways: apply it at arm's length to your finished style to set it for the day, spray onto your fingertips before using your thumb and forefinger to pinch and rub areas of your hair to create a mussed-up texture (this looks great around the hairline on fine flyaways), or spray it onto dry sections of hair before tonging to encourage the curl to stay put for longer. It just does exactly what you want it to – don't bother buying anything else.

DRY SHAMPOO

I think of dry shampoo as a modern woman's hair weapon. Every woman, of every perceivable hair type and colour, can benefit from using dry shampoo. It has gone through a re-branding of sorts in recent years; dry shampoo is no longer used just to refresh dirty hair – it's a fully fledged styling product in its own right. Of course you can use it to absorb excess oil from the scalp, but it's also great for adding volume and texture too. If you have a measly ponytail, try bulking up your hair with a few sprays of dry shampoo and then tying it off into a pony; you'll be surprised just how much thicker it feels. The same technique works if you're creating a topknot, a bun or chignon too.

If you're a dry-shampoo novice be assured that it couldn't be easier to use; just lift your hair in sections and spray the product at the roots underneath. Use your fingers to work the product in a little so that the powder isn't noticeable and remember to keep the can at arm's length from the scalp so that it doesn't clump in one place and look as though you have talcum powder in your hair. I'm not going to reel off a list of brands because to be honest they're all much the same and most still have room for improvement.

JOHN FRIEDA
FRIZZ EASE

If you're trying to create a really sleek style and fighting to get rid of frizz, then John Frieda Frizz Ease is the best solution. Rub a tiny drop (it's very concentrated) between your hands and work through *wet* hair all the way through the lengths and down to the ends. It's just perfect for anyone with a bit of frizz. There's a big misconception that it is designed to make your hair straight, but it doesn't change your natural texture or movement; it just softens frizz, even on wavy or curly hair.

It's quite a watery product so only use it after shampooing and conditioning when your hair is still wet. If you apply Frizz Ease to dry hair you'll make your hair wet again and destroy the style you have just spent ages creating. Any product that's particularly watery in texture should only be applied while the hair itself is still damp, otherwise it will only encourage more frizz.

HERSHESONS
ALMOST EVERYTHING
CREAM

We created our Almost Everything Cream because I am so tired and fed up with the enormity of products thrown at women and want to make life a whole lot simpler. This cream replaces much of the junk on your bathroom shelf; it's not a hairspray or dry shampoo but it's just about everything else. Almost Everything Cream is one of the rare products that can be used on both wet and dry hair, in different ways to achieve different results – *how* you use this product is really important. When you're using a styling product like this it's important to work in layers – just as you do when you're applying your skincare. Don't be tempted to put a huge amount of product into your hair in one go – it will just make your hair look greasy. Add product in increments; work through a pea-sized piece first, then if you need more add another pea-sized piece, and so on. This will allow you to add just the right amount of product for your style whether you're creating something wet-look and sleek or something dishevelled.

Remember, when it comes to most styling products a little goes a long way. If you're using Almost Everything Cream every single day it should still last you a few months at least.

You can use it on wet hair as a leave-in conditioner, serum and a primer by putting a small amount in the palms of your hands and rubbing them together to warm it up and distribute the product before combing it through your hair with your fingers and drying it in. When your hair is dry, work some Almost Everything Cream into it with your fingers for texture, separation, frizz control, condition and shine. If you have very curly and frizzy hair, Almost Everything Cream is the answer, and if you want to create piecey texture just rub it between your hands and create a sandwich (with your hands being the bread and your hair the filling) and pull it down the length of your hair. It's buildable too so you can keep adding and adding until you get to the texture and hold that you want. See, it does almost everything.

COLOR WOW
ROOT COVER UP

This is just a brilliant product. Of course it's good for its intended purpose – which is to temporarily colour or disguise your colour regrowth in between appointments with your colourist – but I love to use it to fill in the hairline. I'll often use it this way with my clients on red-carpet looks where I want the hairline to be a bit fuller, you can really give the impression of thicker hair, which is great when thinning is an issue. If you haven't tried it before, it's a piece of cake; the kit comes with a powder and a short, densely packed brush. Just use the brush to pat the powder onto the root area or around the hairline where things are looking a little sparse. There are eight shades, including a red, so there should be one for you.

TIGI BED HEAD SUPERSTAR
QUEEN FOR A DAY VOLUME SPRAY

I never turn up to a job without this spray in my kit because it is quite literally the business for creating height and volume in hair. It makes hair look thicker and smoother and gives it a long-lasting hold, which is ideal when you're creating some kind of up-do. Most volumising sprays or lotions go very, very sticky in the drying process and this doesn't. Because it's an aerosol it creates a very fine mist so you get guts and hold without reaching a point where you can't put a brush through the hair. You spray it into your hair – even into your roots – while still damp and then blow-dry it in; the volume seems to come out of nowhere. There are other products out there that deliver volume but where I think this particular product excels is in the finish; it doesn't make hair look solid or untouchable, which is quite a feat.

HAIR OIL

Not everyone should use a hair oil – in fact if you have very fine, very limp hair an oil is probably the worst thing you can add into the mix. But hair oils are absolutely great for coarse and curly hair because they replace some of that lost moisture that dehydrated curls are so desperate for, and they add a healthy-looking richness and definition to the shape.

I love to use Kérastase Elixir Ultime, the original Moroccanoil or Phytoelixir Oil on clients with curly hair; if I'm honest, they do much the same thing and deliver almost identical results. The key is to apply the oil while the hair is still wet but the amount you need to use will really depend on how thick and dehydrated your hair is. The easiest thing to do with an oil is to work in layers: express one pump of oil into your palm and rub your hands together to distribute the product (this will help you apply the oil evenly to your hair). Work the oil through your hair from near your roots to your ends or anywhere you feel your hair is particularly parched. If your hair still feels dehydrated work another pump through and so on.

The thicker and coarser your hair, the more oil you will likely need to use but you will know it has had enough when your hair starts to feel softer and more moisturised.

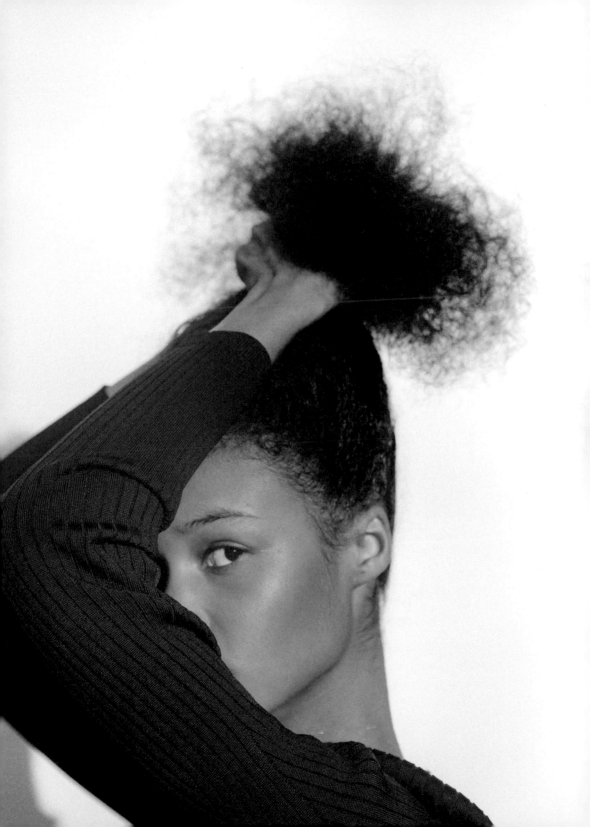

BRUSHES

It's tempting to buy all manner of brushes but regardless of whether your hair is short or long you really only need three in your life. Brushes are really about the *result* you want to achieve rather than your natural hair type and it's for this reason that I have specifically chosen these brushes as they work for everyone.

ROUND-BARRELLED BRUSH

Using a traditional medium-sized round-barrelled brush – like the medium Hershesons Ceramic Ionic Brush – will help you create a smooth and sleek blow dry with a bit of body. The finish is gorgeously luxurious. You want your round brush to be made from synthetic bristles (look for nylon) that create a smoother finish and have a ceramic barrel, which heats up in air-flow from the dryer and 'cooks' the hair from the inside too. We ditched boar bristle in our round brushes at Hershesons about ten to fifteen years ago because they are less effective at helping to smooth or set hair.

MIXED-BRISTLE PADDLE

Think of your mixed-bristle brush as your dressing brush; it's ideal for smoothing the surface of the hair if you're putting it up into a bun, chignon or even a ponytail. Look for a brush containing a mixture of synthetic bristles (such as nylon) and natural (like boar bristles). Mason Pearson are renowned for their mixed-bristle brushes and are well worth a purchase.

DETANGLER

Brushing your hair while it is wet can damage it, yet I know women want to get any knots out before going in with the hairdryer. Try a detangling brush like the Hershesons Knot My Problem Brush, which has gentler bristles and slides through the hair – detangling as it goes – with minimum breakage.

WHEN A BRUSH
WILL NOT DO

The only hair type that requires a slightly different approach is very curly and coily hair, which can be too fragile for a brush. If your hair breaks at the mere mention of a brush, then stick to either a wide-toothed comb or Afro comb and only use it on your hair after you have coated it in a rich mask or pre-shampoo product; this way you can easily (and painlessly) detangle without stressing your hair or scalp.

Remember! Oil, dirt and product build-up can become a breeding ground for bacteria and yeast so it's important to clean your hairbrushes once a month. Soak the brush in warm water and apply some shampoo directly to the bristles, use your hands and fingers to work up a lather and ensure everything is squeaky clean before rinsing and setting it aside to dry. Don't be tempted to speed up the process by putting the brush on a radiator to dry; you may melt the plastic components or the glue holding the bristles in place.

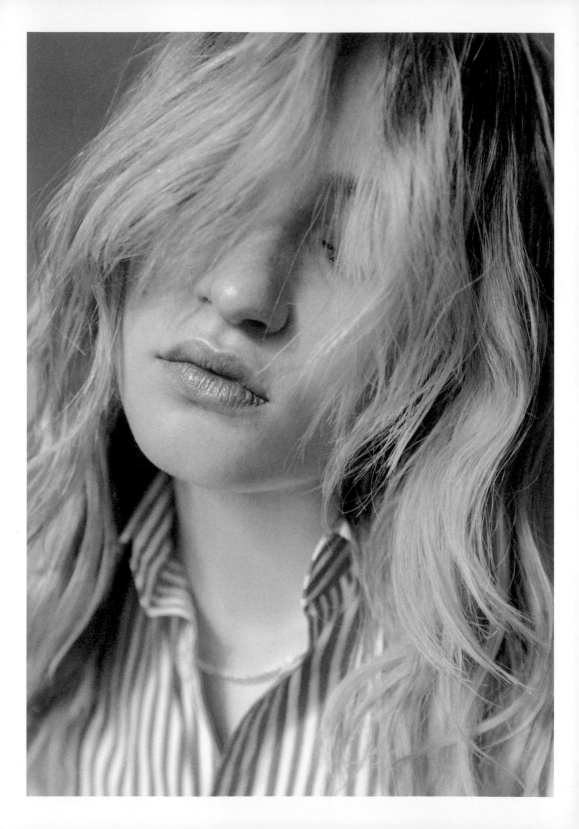

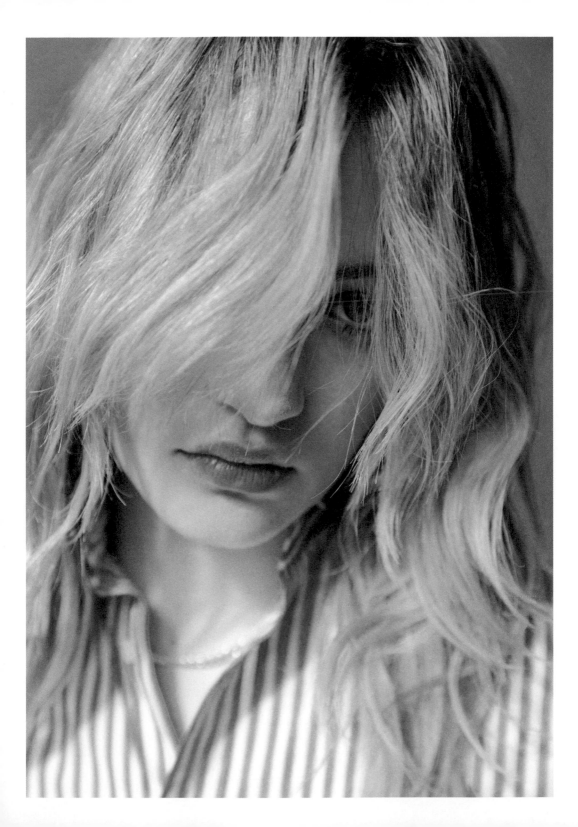

OTHER TOOLS

The tools you use are just as important, if not more important, than the products you use in your hair. There is no need to overcomplicate styling; there certainly are brands that seem to launch a new electrical styling tool every other month but they're not necessarily something you should invest in, or need. I like to keep a tight edit on the tools that I use and while I find a lot of new 'innovations' aren't useful that's not to say they are necessarily bad. There is, however, one exception, I feel; any heated styling tool that suggests it should be used on wet hair (aside from a hairdryer, obviously) is not worth the investment as putting direct heat onto wet hair will just cause a world of damage.

HAIRDRYER

Plenty of women sit in the hairdresser's chair and tell themselves that they can never create the same kind of look at home. They put it down to the skills of the hairdresser, which is flattering, but I can tell you that it's less to do with the stylist and more to do with the hairdryer. Ask yourself, how old is your hairdryer? How much did you spend on it? Plenty of people pick up a bargain hairdryer from the high street, spending maybe £30 maximum in the process (a good hairdryer costs around the £70 mark), and then find that they can't create smooth hairstyles quickly at home.

Your hairdryer choice deserves some research and ultimately you're looking for two things: speed and heat. Great hairdryers are those that hit the sweet spot between the two; lots of speed without heat is ineffective, but too much heat and you can burn your scalp. You need a hairdryer that has a cool-to-hot temperature and slow-to-fast speed so you can select them for yourself. These two things have to be in sync and unfortunately that doesn't always come cheap, but while a decent hairdryer can seem somewhat of an expense just consider how often you use it and how many years you hang on to it. Thinking about it, it's a veritable steal.

Follow these rules and never fall foul to a bad hairdryer ever again:

Ignore any number that makes up the brand name: They may call themselves a 3,000, or a 4,000, but that doesn't necessarily translate to the wattage so read the spec.

Try before you buy: This is so important. You're likely to keep a hairdryer for some time so you need to know that it serves your purposes. Go to a shop like John Lewis where you can try a display model, and get a feel for the heat and speed, before putting down cash.

Don't be swept up by the design: When Dyson launched its Supersonic hairdryer everyone went potty for it without stopping to check that it actually delivers. It *is* on the quiet side, which I concede is useful when you're drying your hair early in the morning and you're mindful not to wake everyone in the house, but in my opinion, it greatly falls short of that aforementioned sweet spot and is not ideal for anyone with any kind of frizz or irregular texture. The truth is, expectations are low when it comes to hairdryers, so – in my opinion – the Dyson in comparison to many others looks good but if you want to reduce frizz and create a decent smooth blow dry then I just don't think it delivers. The point I'm making is, don't allow yourself to get caught up in marketing hype; research, read reviews and remember, try before you buy.

Consider attachments: There are really only two attachments you could possibly need, and it's unlikely that you'll need both. Most hairdryers come with a nozzle that allows you to concentrate the airflow in one place and create a smoother finish. If you like to wear your hair curly you will really benefit from a diffuser attachment, which holds your hair in place in a kind of dish as it circulates air around the curls. There was a time when most hairdryers came with a diffuser attachment but they have fallen out of fashion in the last few years and now most of them don't – many manufacturers do sell them separately though. There's a brilliant diffuser that we use a lot backstage; it's called the Ion Mesh Diffuser by YS Park (you can find it on sessionkit.com) which is a brilliant update on a traditional diffuser and because it is made out of fabric it can attach to any hairdryer.

CURLING TONG

There's no need to own multiple tongs of all shapes and sizes – one will do just fine. The size of the barrel defines the size of the curl, so for a tight and defined curl a small barrel is in order, and for something loose and wavier, a larger barrel is needed. I always use the Hershesons Tourmaline Professional Curling Tong. It has a 2.5-centimetre barrel, which I think is the optimum size for creating nicely relaxed waves whether your hair is bob length or long. You'll notice that some tongs come with a clamp and others do not. The end result is the same whether you use a clamp or not; however, using a clamp takes a little practice.

So you might wonder why you would bother with a clamp at all in that case. If your hair has been chemically treated in any way – whether we're talking permanent straightening, perming or colour – the outer cuticles have already been lifted and so heat penetrates the hair pretty quickly. Essentially, this means that it doesn't take much work to get a curl or wave to set into the hair. But if your hair is practically virgin, if the texture and colour are both natural, then the cuticle is likely to still be intact, which means it's going to take a bit more effort to get the same wave or curl. A clamp allows you to squash the hair onto the barrel and heat the hair from both sides so you can create a curl.

If you're new to this and you are not adept at tonging I would suggest using a tong without a clamp as they are so much easier to get to grips with.

CERAMIC STRAIGHTENERS

Thankfully, straightening irons have come a long way from their clunky origins and are virtually unrecognisable from their predecessor, which, in all honesty, just didn't work at all. I first really cottoned on to straighteners in the late nineties. I was an assistant on a shoot for Italian *Vogue* and there was a hairdresser who was using these big, clumpy industrial irons that got the hair super-straight. So, back home I decided to start importing straighteners so women in the UK could get that perfectly ironed finish too. I remember seeing a piece in *Allure* magazine on Eugene Souleiman creating poker-straight hair at Prada. It was such a new thing then and everybody went mad for it.

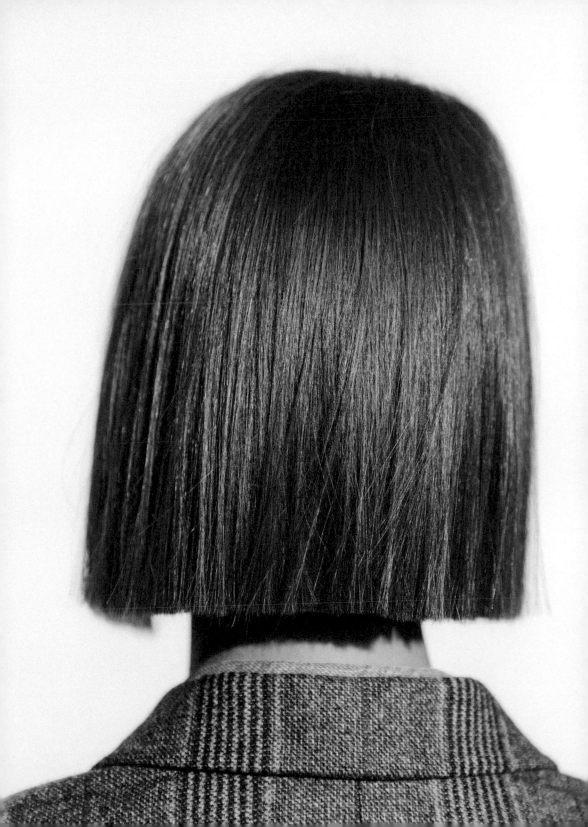

When irons first came out they were the only thing that could give you poker-straight ends but actually nowadays we use straightening irons to do lots of other things apart from just make hair straight. You can use a straightening iron to get a bit of a kink or a bit of a bend, you can plait your hair and run your irons over it to set in a bit of slept-in wave, or you can use the irons to take out too prom-style ringlets. Their usage has evolved over the years and that's what should make them a staple in your kit.

Brands come and go but the technology speaks for itself. Ceramic plates warm up evenly so you get an equal distribution of heat throughout the hair, while titanium plates won't drag or snag and they create an impossibly smooth, mirror-like finish. I know that there are some of you who will insist on using your straightening irons every day, and I know there is nothing I can do to persuade you to do otherwise – but be aware that even if you're using a heat-protection product you cannot completely defend your hair against damage. Applying heat directly to the hair ultimately wears down the protective cuticle and corrupts the cortex of the hair, which gives it its strength. This results in dry and rough hair that looks frizzy and is prone to breakage.

If you can scale back your usage to every other day (or two or three times a week) then you will be shielding your hair from a whole lot of mayhem. If, however, you resolutely stand by using your straighteners every day, be prepared to get the ends cut regularly, have split ends snipped away and make sure you're using strengthening protein-packed intensive masks every week.

FINGERS

Your hands and fingers are quite possibly the best styling tool available to you; don't overlook them. It's easy to get swept up with new and promising brush designs that claim to deliver everything under the sun – and yes, as you've already read, there are a few brushes that I think are non-negotiable – but that's not to say that they replace your fingers. Hairstylists use their hands far more than they do their tools, and one in particular, Christiaan Houtenbos (who also happens to be one of the most respected stylists in the biz) has a reputation for turning up on-set with a tiny kit because he creates everything with his hands. Your hands are your best tools for distributing product throughout your hair and creating root-lift and soft bed-hair texture, so don't forget them.

Here are just some of the things you can do without a brush regardless of your hair type:

Create movement and separation: You can create the most beautiful texture just by rubbing pieces of hair from the roots to the ends between your thumb and forefinger. It's something you will always see a great stylist do. If you're wearing your hair up in a pony or a bun, this is a great technique for softening the hairline and preventing everything from looking too angular and neat.

Get relaxed ends: It's easy to achieve slept-in dishevelled ends just by rubbing hair between the palms of your hands.

Teasing: You really don't need a comb or brush to tease your hair or create height. Use your fingers as a comb to grip your hair in sections and push it back on itself at the root. The volume is far softer than you get with a brush and it's easier to comb out afterwards.

Create waves: There are two ways to do this without having to pick up a brush or a tong. Section out your hair while it is still damp and fold the section up towards your scalp – in a kind of concertina – and then pin in place while everything dries. The other tried-and-tested method for a softer, looser wave is to simply twist sections around your fingers as your hair dries.

Natural volume: Throw your head upside down when you're blow-drying and use your hands to push and pull your hair away from you. When you flick your head back you'll have more volume than you'll know what to do with.

Tame frizz: Use your fingers like a comb to grip and gently pull your hair at the roots while you're drying it. You can get rid of maybe 60 to 70 per cent of your frizz just by doing this simple movement and that's before even touching a brush or a pair of straightening irons.

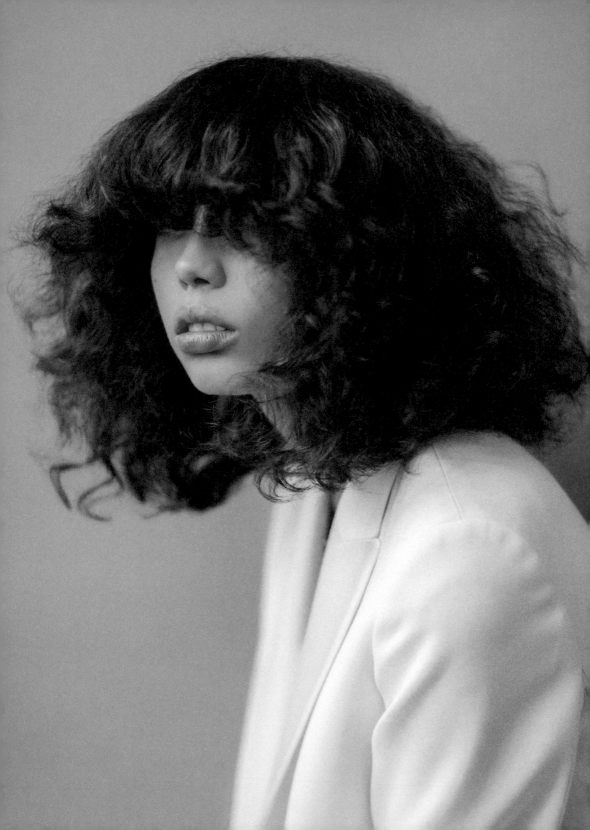

YOUR
HAIR
ROUTINE

'Never be caught
without great hair
ever again'

Forget what magazines tell you about shampoo, condition, blow dry and straighten. The rules have changed and a modern haircare and styling routine is far from a one-size-fits-all approach. Clean hair, lovely though it may feel, isn't always the best for styling, and some styles simply look better without interminable fussing in the drying process. Do you need to wear a hair primer? Sometimes. Do you know when and where to apply it? Possibly not. This is what constitutes a sound haircare routine; follow this to the T and never be caught without great hair ever again.

STEP 1
PRE-POO (OPTIONAL)

I agree with what you're thinking: this sounds like an utterly undesirable thing to do to your hair and whoever initially came up with the name of it has some explaining to do. If you're not familiar with pre-pooing, it's essentially a pre-shampoo treatment designed to detangle, hydrate and strengthen your hair.

If you have very curly, coily or Afro hair you're probably already doing this – or you've at least heard of it – but this method has similar benefits for less curly, wavy and straight hair types too. Pre-pooing works exceptionally well with coils and Afro, as the tighter the coil the drier the hair tends to be.

To pre-poo you just need to section out your hair with your finger or a comb, and work through your pre-poo product of choice. A great pre-poo product is oily, rich and nourishing. Coconut oil, or a hair oil like Moroccanoil, are both great options. Philip Kingsley's Elasticizer (originally created for Audrey Hepburn when she complained that the constant styling on-set was wrecking her hair) contains hydrolysed elastin, castor oil, olive oil and glycerine and makes for a brilliant pre-shampoo treatment as it cleanses away dirt and product build-up without stressing the scalp.

Once fully coated, cover your hair with a shower cap and leave it to do its thing for at least twenty minutes, preferably longer, or even overnight. Then shampoo out. If you have very coarse, curly or Afro hair you may use this method of cleansing every time you wash your hair; alternatively, incorporate it into your routine once every other week.

STEP 2

SHAMPOO

'How often should I wash my hair?' It's a question I am always asked by clients and beauty journalists. Unfortunately, there isn't a straightforward answer. Some trichologists recommend that you wash your hair every day as you would your face. And I get it, your scalp goes everywhere your face does and you wouldn't think of going a whole day without washing that. However, it's just not feasible for some women to wash their hair every day. For starters, if you have a job and a family it can be a near-impossible task to find time in the morning to wash and dry your hair.

Secondly, some women have hair that refuses to behave when it is washed every day; perhaps it becomes too dehydrated, your scalp may be too sensitive and your hair may be unruly. If you have very coily or Afro hair you may only want to wash your hair once a week because the curlier the hair, the drier it tends to be naturally, which is only exacerbated by washing it. It's not advisable to leave it more than a week, however, because if dirt and oils are allowed to accumulate they will stress your scalp.

If you have Afro hair and find that shampoo has only ever dried your hair out even further, then you may be better off just pre-pooing or co-washing (more on this next); this won't achieve the same level of clean but it will cleanse your hair sufficiently without stripping it of its natural oils and turning it into an unmanageable wiry mess.

Lastly, from a styling point of view, with the exception of curly hair, it is actually easier to style hair when it is not freshly washed; it has a little more guts and holds a style better when it isn't so clean. So it's your call – wash your hair as frequently as you feel the need to.

One thing I do insist on, however, is that when you *do* wash your hair, you wash it twice. Double Cleansing as a method has been a trend in skincare for a while now and the principles are the same when it comes to your hair. Your first clean will remove surface dirt and product and your second cleanse will really penetrate and do a deep clean. There's no need for two separate shampoos; use the same product. We're all familiar with how to shampoo: rinse your hair thoroughly (this step will remove some dirt before you've even touched the shampoo bottle), work your shampoo over your scalp and down to your ends and massage it in with your fingertips. This massage will stimulate your scalp and help to remove any dead skin that may have collected on the surface and in hair follicles. Rinse and repeat a second time with warm water and move on to condition.

CO-WASH

As I mentioned, if when you were reading What's your Hair Type? you identified yourself as an extremely curly, coily or Afro hair type, then shampooing just may not work for you. Shampoos by design lift oils from the hair, but as a very curly hair type you have little oil to begin with. This often means that shampooing – even only once a week – can leave your hair feeling parched, coarse and unmanageable. Pre-pooing with coconut oil or a hair oil works for many women who want to clean their Afro without destroying the texture, but some find it a little too heavy. Co-washing is the alternative and essentially means skipping the shampoo and cleansing with conditioner only.

Cleansing with just a conditioner will not get you to that squeaky-clean stage, but it does contain trace amounts of detergent (look for cetrimonium and behentrimonium chloride on the ingredients list to be sure) so you will remove some dirt *and* keep your hair hydrated and easier to manage. You can use a regular conditioner or try some of the newer co-washing products in the shops, which go big on conditioning oils like marula and sweet almond oil and contain cleansing ingredients that won't dry your curls out. Vernon François Co-Wash Shampoo, Living Proof Curl Conditioning Wash, Bouclème Curl Cleanser, Charlotte Mensah Manketti Oil Shampoo and Mizani Cream Cleansing Conditioner are all brilliant and inexpensive. There's no right or wrong here – you just have to try it and see if it works for you.

Co-washing is easy and doesn't require an ounce of skill to pull off. Rinse your hair in the shower, and once it is fully saturated divide it into sections using your fingers and apply your conditioning product from the scalp to

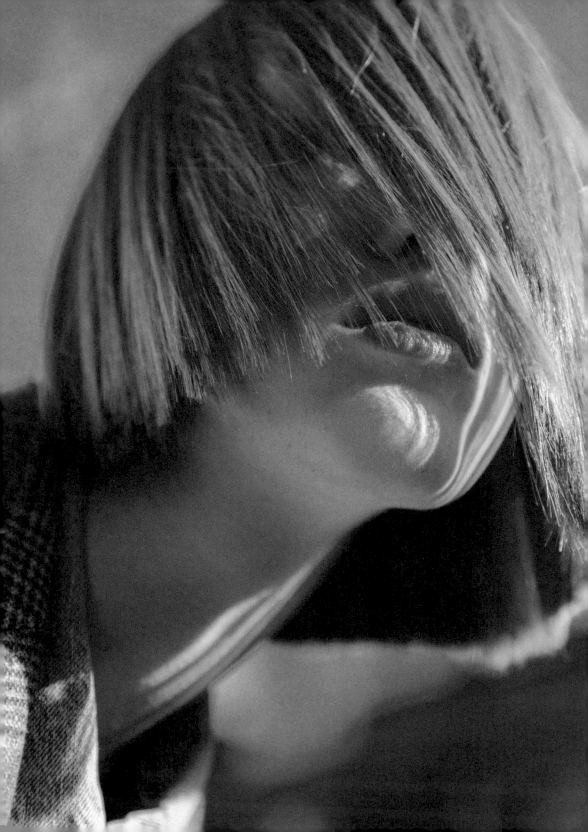

the ends. I know it sounds unusual to put conditioner on your scalp but remember, in this instance you're using it to cleanse your hair too and your scalp absolutely needs cleaning regularly. Work the product through your hair and over your scalp as you would a shampoo but don't expect any suds or foam – conditioners do not contain the sulphates that are present in shampoos so there won't be such a dramatic display. If your hair is very knotty, now is a good time to detangle using a wide-toothed comb. Then rinse thoroughly.

STEP 3

CONDITION

On the whole, unless you have very curly, coily or Afro hair, your hair benefits from conditioning after you shampoo. Shampoo raises the hair's cuticle in order to lift away dirt, which can leave hair looking fluffy and coarse. The role of the conditioner is to swoop in and smooth the cuticle again so that hair looks shiny and feels silkier. There is more than a cosmetic function to conditioner, though; while your cuticle remains open your hair is in a weak and vulnerable position and susceptible to damage from the environment and heat styling. When you close off that cuticle you're battening down the hatches against aggressors. Conditioners are especially important if you have had any kind of chemical treatment such as a perm, permanent straightening or even colour; all of these treatments raise your cuticle layer and it's essential to remedy that.

While shampoo, to some extent, is a one-size-fits-all kind of product (after all, the sole purpose of a shampoo is really just to remove dirt), conditioner can be far more prescriptive. Make sure you're buying a product that is suitable for your needs. Thankfully, you don't have to be a chemist to decipher the labels and find the right conditioner for your hair. Just look at the front of the bottle to see which concern it addresses but don't get too weighed down with outlandish claims and pseudo-science – see them for what they are, which is some heavy-handed marketing. Look through the fluff to its most basic claims; essentially you just need to know whether it's hydrating, repairing, thickening, smoothing etc.

Hydration: If your hair feels coarse and looks rough it will need moisture so be sure to buy a conditioner that says it's hydrating or moisture-boosting, and look for ingredients such as fatty alcohols and moisturisers like glycerine and shea butter.

Repairing: Hair broken and splitting? Then it's damaged. Look for conditioners that say they're repairing, strengthening and rebuilding, to shore up your defences.

Frizz taming: Conditioners that are marketed for frizzy hair contain ingredients that guard against humidity so that it's less likely to puff up during the day.

Thickening: All conditioners make hair flat, right? Wrong. Body-building conditioners use ingredients like hydrolysed wheat proteins to bulk out strands. The label should direct you towards its purpose, but checking the ingredients list for these will help too.

It's easy to assume that everyone knows how to condition their hair but if the number of women who complain to me that their conditioner weighs their hair down is anything to go by, a fair few people are still getting it wrong. Thoroughly rinse away every trace of shampoo, squeeze some of the water out of your hair, pour a small amount of conditioner into the palm of your hand (the amount will depend on the length of your hair but you should aim for a blob around the size of a 50p piece), rub your hands together to distribute the product and then work it through your mid-lengths and ends. Unless co-washing, do not apply conditioner to your roots! It is the ultimate no-no. Your roots receive plenty of oils from your scalp so you do not need extra hydration or condition here. If you decide to ignore my advice, be prepared to kiss goodbye to volume and say hello to greasy hair.

If your hair is very knotty, use this time to detangle with a wide-toothed comb or the Hershesons Knot My Problem brush, which will slip through and disperse knots without damaging your hair. Whenever you are combing your hair while it is wet, always work from the bottom and make your way up your hair only once you have cleared any knots in your way. Your hair is vulnerable to damage when it is wet and this is the only way of clearing tangles without overly stressing your hair.

Conditioner doesn't need to be left on for very long to do its thing – a few seconds max – so be quick about washing it out. Be thorough with this rinse to ensure every trace of conditioner is gone. If any remains it will be tricky to style your hair and it will begin to feel very greasy very quickly.

STEP 4
HAIR MASK (OPTIONAL)

Some people just can't get on board with a hair mask – and that's okay – but there are others who swear by them. A good mask goes beyond a conditioner; they contain heavier conditioning ingredients like oils and butters, plus quats (a family of conditioning ingredients skilled at detangling) and wax-based conditioners, so they are very nourishing and very hydrating (which is precisely why some women with extremely fine hair will never be convinced to use a mask – and I don't blame them).

If you have medium to thick hair that's straight, wavy, curly or coarse, then using a mask once or twice a week is a brilliant idea. The conditioners work a little harder so your hair looks and feels stronger, glossier and smoother – which is no bad thing. Try not to use a hair mask more than twice a week as this could only serve to weigh your hair down.

When you are using a mask, use it in place of your conditioner not on top of it. Apply a generous amount through your mid-lengths and ends (making sure to thoroughly cover your ends as they are the oldest and most worn part of your hair), twist your hair up onto the top of your head and don a shower cap. The heat produced by your scalp will be trapped inside the cap and encourage the mask to work even harder. Leave the product on for as long as the directions stipulate and then thoroughly wash it out with warm water. Be sure to remove every trace of your mask so as not to weigh your hair down later.

Choose your mask in exactly the same way you do your conditioner; ask yourself what are your first and second hair concerns in terms of priority, and look for a mask that addresses one or both of them.

TOWEL-DRY

You're out of the shower, you're shivering and dripping wet and you're tempted to start drying your hair straight away if only to warm up. But wait. You need to remove some of the water from your hair before you do anything else; this will speed up your drying time considerably.

Towel-drying sounds fairly easy but it can be barbaric if done incorrectly. Do not just grab your bath towel and have at it; scrubbing, yanking and buffing your hair with a regular towel will damage your hair and lift its cuticle so that it dries in a cloud of frizz and flyaways. Approach your hair gently, and with a microfibre towel. These are far from glamorous but they do an admirable job of starting the drying process without massacring your hair; they absorb water much quicker than a regular towel and thanks to the way they are woven they are far less aggressive with your precious hair.

Lightly pat water from your hair with your microfibre towel, then use it to twist your hair up into a turban and leave it that way until you are ready to blow-dry. Microfibre towels are inexpensive and can be found in most stores, but there are, of course, some brands – such as Aquis and Bouclème – that specifically make them for your hair.

STEP 6
COMB AND APPLY PRODUCT

Now you're ready to get cracking. Don't use a normal brush on your hair while it is wet as this is when it is most vulnerable to damage. Instead, use a wide-toothed comb or Hershesons Knot My Problem brush to gently work through any tangles.

Next, apply some Almost Everything Cream. I think this is the first step for every single hair type, from fine and straight, to coarse, curly and Afro, and from dry to greasy. Put a small amount into one palm and then rub both palms together to spread the product. Many women make the mistake of putting the product into their hand and then transferring it straight to their hair – it's essential to rub your hands together first so that you get an even coating on your hair. If your hair dries clumpy I'm willing to bet it's because

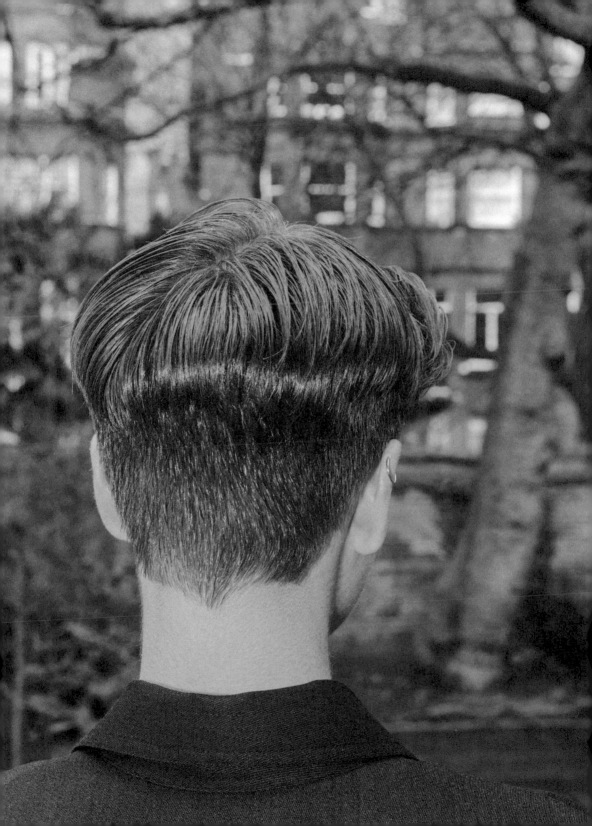

you're not getting this step right. Now use your hands like a comb and work it through your hair. This step will prep your hair for heat, strengthen and nourish, smooth and reduce frizz and take down some of the fluffiness that comes with freshly washed hair and makes it difficult to style. Alternatively, apply a styling cream that contains heat protection.

If your frizz is particularly irate and you want a smooth final result, now is also the time to use some John Frieda Frizz Ease. Frizz Ease is potent stuff so you only need a very small amount. Apply it to your hair while it is still wet by working it first in between your hands and then through your mid-lengths and ends. Do not apply it near your roots.

If you're air-drying there's not really anything else you need to do except twist a few sections of hair around a finger to encourage a little movement. But if you're now going to move on to a hairdryer and maybe an iron or tong, then you need to add some additional heat protection. Heated styling tools reach staggeringly high temperatures in order to fix your hair into a new shape, but unfortunately that same heat can damage the outer cuticle layer of your hair and wreak havoc with its cortex. L'Oréal Professionnel Tecni.Art Constructor and Philip Kingsley Daily Damage Defence are both brilliantly able heat protectors. Mist either one over your entire hair, roots to ends, basically anywhere that is going to be touched by the heat.

STEP 7
DRY

BLOW-DRY
Let's be honest, most women spend less than five minutes in front of the mirror, with their hairdryer temperature on full whack, blasting their hair in every direction imaginable only to throw everything down in a hump, proclaim their hair looks shit, and give up. Sound familiar? I know that blow-drying your hair sucks – there are far more pleasurable pursuits in life – but isn't great hair worth a little time and effort? You don't need to be a trained professional to dry your hair properly and make it look halfway decent. Follow these *simple* steps and you'll never again feel the urge to curse your hair.

Protect: Before you even lay a finger on your hairdryer remember to properly protect your hair with a heat-defence product.

Rough-dry: Don't be tempted to begin drying your hair with a hairbrush. While your hair is still wet it's very vulnerable to damage and a brush is about as damaging as it gets. Start your hairdryer on a low heat and speed setting and rough-dry your hair – using just your hands – until your hair is about 95 per cent dry. Then, and only then, should you use a brush. Skipping the brush for the first part doesn't just minimise damage, it stops you from wasting your time because your hair needs to be almost dry before you can begin shaping it properly.

If you're worried about what not using a brush will do for your frizz, don't: you can eliminate much of the fluff with just your hands. This rough-drying technique is actually just as much about styling as it is about drying and it can shorten your overall styling time by about half.

Honing your style: If you're creating something with lots of volume or something very sleek then you should start using a brush only once your hair is almost entirely dry. The right brush depends on the look you want to create. For something voluminous, full-bodied and luxurious, use a round-barrelled brush; wrap your hair in sections around the brush and blast it in a downwards direction with your hairdryer (the nozzle of your hairdryer should be parallel to the brush), then remove the heat and allow the hair to cool slightly around the bristles before letting it down. But you don't always have to use a brush and, in fact, I hardly ever use a brush any more. I think it is better to rough-dry your hair and then use a tong or an iron to get it into the style you want – neither of which require a brush.

My wife has a brilliant technique when it comes to her hair. She rough-dries it and then she flicks her hair back and forth a couple of times, then flings it forward over her head so it's all falling in the same direction. Then she just ties it up into a loose bun, and leaves it alone for a bit to set before letting it down. And it just looks amazing. I'm not one for hair looking too manicured, and air-drying is a great antidote to manicured hair. It looks kind of Parisian, very easy and nonchalant.

Use your hands: As a hairdresser I rely on my hands a great deal more than I do a brush. You can tackle so much of your styling by using your hands in the rough-drying process during those first couple of minutes. To soften a cowlick you should use your fingers like a comb to grab and pull your hair taut while it is still wet to smooth oddities. You *can* use a round-barrelled brush to do this if you're particularly skilled but I just don't think it's necessary. Similarly, you can reduce the appearance of frizz with the same technique; keep the hair taut and the airflow from your hairdryer pointed downwards in the direction you want your hair to fall.

Create volume: There's a formula for volume, and it's a very simple one: wherever you point the airflow from your dryer is where you will create body and lift. Get the nozzle of your dryer up close to the roots of your hair – if that's where you want to see some volume – and use your hands to pull your hair from side to side in opposite directions to lift it away from your scalp. It's this action that creates lift and hails back to my dad's mantra to live by that 'every movement must have a meaning'.

Create shine and minimise frizz: In order for your hair to look shiny you must encourage your cuticle layer to lie flat. Make sure your hairdryer is fitted with a nozzle to concentrate the air in one place and keep the direction of airflow skimming down the hair shaft. Don't lose your patience and start drying your hair in every which way otherwise you risk creating more frizz. Keeping the airflow in the right direction helps to eliminate tangles and force the cuticle layer to lie neatly – this in turn softens frizz and maximises light reflection and shine.

Freshly washed hair, while undeniably lovely, tends to be quite soft and fluffy, and not so easy to style. It's why you always hear hairdressers talking about 'day 2' hair. If your hair *is* freshly washed and drying on the fluffy side, just add another drop of styling cream, about the size of a 2p piece, rub it into your hands and scrunch it into your hair. It will give some guts to the strands and take down some of the fluff.

Create defined and bouncy curls: It's time to bring the diffuser out of the eighties. It is rather brilliant for quickly drying your curls and adding definition

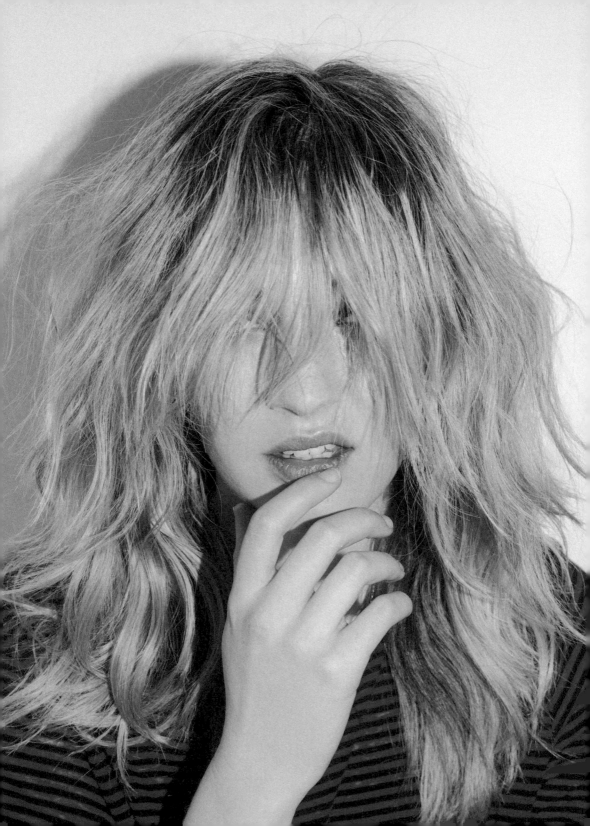

and bounce because it allows air to circulate around the hair. There was a time when hairdryers typically came with a diffuser attachment and while that's not always the case now it is easily rectified; just go to the website for the company that made your dryer and order the diffuser separately. Or try the fabric diffuser by YS Park that you can attach to any hairdryer.

Once your attachment is fitted in place, hold your dryer with the diffuser facing upwards and pool your hair (do not allow it to actually touch your scalp) – one section at a time – into the basin. Two things to remember: handle your hair gently so as not to disturb your curl pattern and leave your hair in the diffuser for as long as it takes for it to dry completely.

Keep going: Women tend to lose patience with their hair and not allow it long enough to dry. But allowing yourself just another couple of minutes will make all the difference to the finish of your hair. Think about it: you spend two or three minutes cleaning your teeth in the morning, and that's all the extra time I'm asking for – not half an hour, just another couple of minutes. If you finish while there is still some moisture left, your hair will not stay in shape and it will frizz and puff up at the slightest provocation. You still don't need to use a brush at this point, your hands are perfectly capable of doing the job. Dry your hair until it is *completely* dry.

To finish: Once your hair is totally dry, give it a final blast of cold air from your hairdryer to lock the cuticle in position and ramp up the shine. Keep the airflow facing down the hair shaft so as not to cause it to frizz at the last hurdle.

AIR-DRY

There was a time when women wouldn't even consider allowing their hair to dry naturally because it would mean showing the world their natural texture. As if that was something to be ashamed of. Now, thankfully, the tables have turned and women are celebrating things that make them unique and stand out from the crowd, and their hair – whether it's curly, or irregularly kinked, or poker straight – is all part of that.

If you have a little bit of natural movement and want to enhance it ever so slightly without using a tong, air-drying is a brilliant option. Once you have worked through your styling cream just twist sections around your finger to encourage some shape and tuck a few bits behind your ears so they take on an impression. Then let nature do its thing.

You don't always have to dry your hair with a hairdryer and you may find that washing your hair at night and tying it up while it dries is a better use of your time. Stylist Christiaan Houtenbos often ties hair up into two or three nineties-esque Space Buns – or Baby Spice buns – so that the hair dries with movement and texture without the use of heat.

PLOP

Another ridiculous name for a remarkably clever technique. Where on earth do people get these names from? Plopping is a fantastic way of drying curls without heat. Heat styling inevitably draws some moisture out of the hair and, as curls are naturally dry anyway, this can be somewhat problematic. Once you have applied your wet-styling products such as Almost Everything Cream or John Frieda's Frizz Ease, just lay your towel (microfibre, remember – never use a normal bath towel on your hair) on a table in front of you, then bend forward so your head is upside down and your hair 'plops' into the centre of the towel. You want to make sure your hair is all falling in one direction.

Grab the end of the towel closest to your face and bring the two sides together to meet at the nape of your neck, then bring the opposite side up and over your head to meet them.

Lastly, gather the two sides of towel that are left either side of your head and bring them together behind your head and tuck them in. All the while, be conscious of not flattening your curls. It sounds like an almighty faff but trust me, it is a lot simpler than it sounds and once you have tried it a couple of times you'll have the technique down. If you're still unsure, there are literally thousands of videos on YouTube demonstrating the technique.

Once your curls are safely ensconced in your microfibre towel you can go about your business, or even go to bed, and all you have to do once you let your hair down is separate the curls with your fingers. This technique should ensure that your curls are both defined and frizz free. And you didn't even need to look sideways at a diffuser.

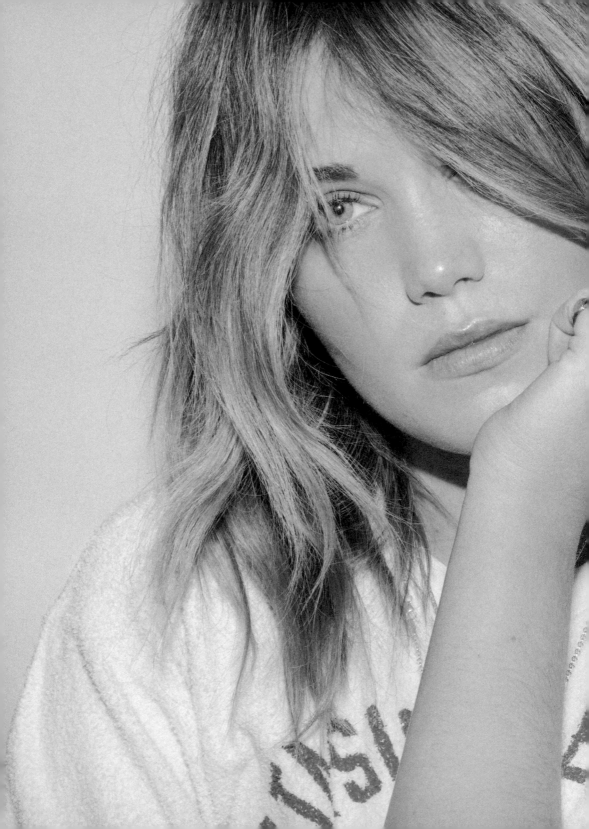

STEP 8
HEAT STYLING

Never use curling tongs or straightening irons on wet hair; you will boil the moisture within the hair shaft and make it blister, causing irrevocable damage. Follow the previous instructions concerning applying heat protection and drying your hair until it is *completely* dry. If you can hear a cracking or snapping sound as you pass your straighteners over your hair then you still have moisture in there and you should stop and pick up your hairdryer again. Only once you have eliminated every drop of water from your hair should you plug in your heated styling tool. Then you can go about creating your style.

If you're straightening your hair it can help to have a mirror both in front of you and behind so you can see the back of your head. Straighteners, naturally, get very hot and can cause damage despite your diligent use of a heat protector. Aim to go over a section only twice (once if you can get away with it) but the plates need to be in contact with your hair long enough to create shape, so while you're only going over that section once or twice, you're really making each pass of the iron count.

If you're curling or waving your hair use a medium-sized barrelled tong (about 2.5 centimetres in diameter) and start tonging your hair from the top of your head and around the outer layers of your hair, slowly working your way to the back of your head. For a relaxed and modern curl, leave a couple of centimetres of root and ends out of the tong so that they are less wavy than the rest of your hair, and don't worry if you miss a few sections; in my opinion, curls and waves look so much better when they're not uniform.

STEP 9
FINISH

It's time to put your hands to good use again. If you have created a wave or a curl, use your fingers to separate out the strands and rough up the texture a little. Use your forefinger and thumb to pinch and rub your hair in places to make whatever style you have created look a little more relaxed. Elnett is a must. Keep the can at arm's length so that you can veil your hair in a light and even mist.

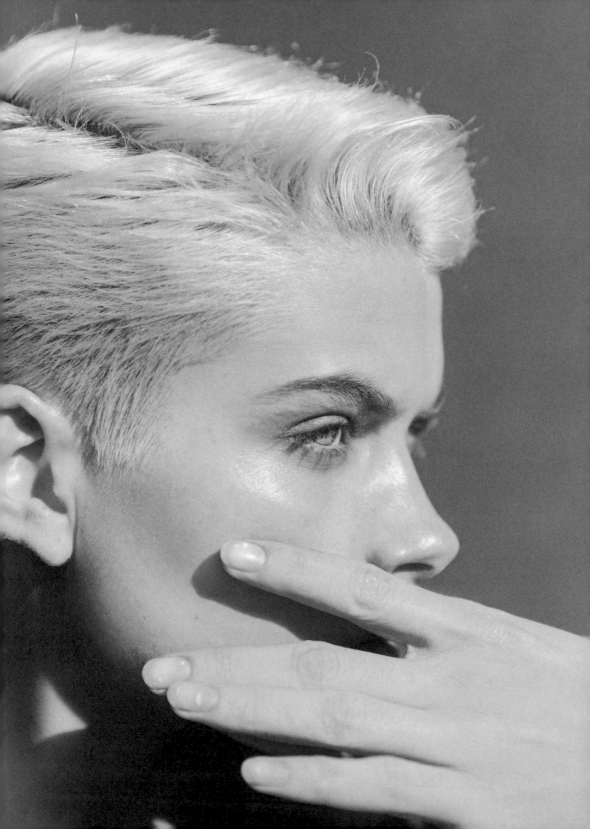

RULES

ARE

THERE

TO

BE

BROKEN

'Don't let
anyone
tell you
no'

If you were to log on to our website right now (Hershesons.com) you would see a kind of mission statement on the first page you come to. It says, 'We don't believe in limits, boundaries or rules.' And we live by it.

There are far too many limits imposed on us in the real world; let's not extend that to hair also. We've torn up the rule book when it comes to the way you're 'technically' meant to cut hair and you'll never hear one of our stylists or colourists use confusing jargon or hairdresser talk. We want to cut the crap from hairdressing and styling and give it to you straight.

RULES WORTH BREAKING

Some common hair beliefs are, quite frankly, completely irrelevant for the way we live our lives now. Personal style is so much more important than following pre-prescribed trends and rules.

~~SHORT HAIR IS FOR TOMBOYS AND OLDER LADIES~~

Utter tosh. The idea that long hair is feminine and short hair is boyish is just complete rubbish. The space we're occupying in history is exciting because women (and men) are challenging outdated gender myths such as these. Who cares if you wear your hair short or long? That's a personal decision only you can make. I can't imagine that you would allow a backwards stereotype to influence you. Besides, nowhere is it written that short hair can't be beautiful and/or sexy.

~~WOMEN OVER FORTY SHOULD CUT THEIR HAIR~~

Try telling that to Julianne Moore and Julia Roberts, both of whom are in their fifties and look absolutely incredible with long hair. The length of your hair has everything to do with your own sense of personal style and how you like to wear your hair, and absolutely nothing to do with the year you were born. 'Age' means something very different now from what it once did, and thankfully more and more women are not allowing their age to become a factor when deciding how to wear their hair. An eighteen- and an eighty-year-old should be able to have the same haircut, you should be able to rock the same vibe. You may just need to adapt how to style it. Age doesn't define you.

~~GREYS SHOULD BE DYED~~

If you wish to dye your greys that is entirely up to you but no one should feel that it is expected of them. Grey hair can do wonderful things for your skin tone and it makes you stand out from the crowd. Sarah Harris of British *Vogue* proves beyond doubt that grey hair can be fashionable and modern. Fashion designer Jenna Lyons (formerly of J.Crew) has been a long-term brunette but over the last year or so she has allowed her grey hairs to creep through. Now almost the entire front section is a shocking shade of white and it looks so stylish. Should you wish to embrace your greys too, more power to you.

~~DARK BROWS SHOULD NEVER BE SEEN ON BLONDES~~

I, for one, think darker brows look great on blondes. Blonde brows can sometimes get a little lost amongst other facial features and introducing a darker shade to them (whether with a semi-permanent tint or make-up) can bring focus and definition to your whole eye area. Slightly (keyword, slightly – extremes can be less palatable) darker brows will become part of your own unique sense of style. Just look at Cara Delevingne: her combination of dark brows and lighter hair has become her trademark.

CURLS ARE NOT OFFICE APPROPRIATE

Sadly, curls have been persecuted for a very long time. Tight coils and Afro hair have, in the past, earned a reputation for being too laid-back and not professional enough, which is utterly crazy. Your hair is part of your image, it's part of the message you're putting out into the world, and I don't think an employer in any field has the right (or the expertise) to say whether that message falls beyond the boundaries of professionalism. Thankfully, I don't think there are many companies that try to pull this crap any more because the moment anyone tries to they're often shamed – deservedly so – on social media and in the papers.

DARK ROOTS ARE A TOTAL FAUX PAS

Maybe at one point in time that was true but this is certainly not the case now. Modern colour techniques like balayage deliberately make the root area dark and the ends lighter both to make hair look more natural and to soften regrowth. If you think about natural colour, the roots are always half a shade or a shade darker than the rest of the hair so recreating that with a bottled colour lends more credibility to the end result. A solid all-over colour can look flat and uninteresting. But play with the depth of your colour in places – like your roots – and your hair very quickly becomes something more. I don't think this is a short-lived trend, I think hair colour has evolved.

YOU SHOULD GET A FRINGE TO HIDE YOUR WRINKLES

What nonsense. You should only ever get a fringe because you really want a fringe. Lines and wrinkles are not shameful and – while you can hide them if you want – there's no rule that says they have to be hidden. If you *do* want to address your lines, your money is better spent in the pursuit of great skincare and a brilliant aesthetician.

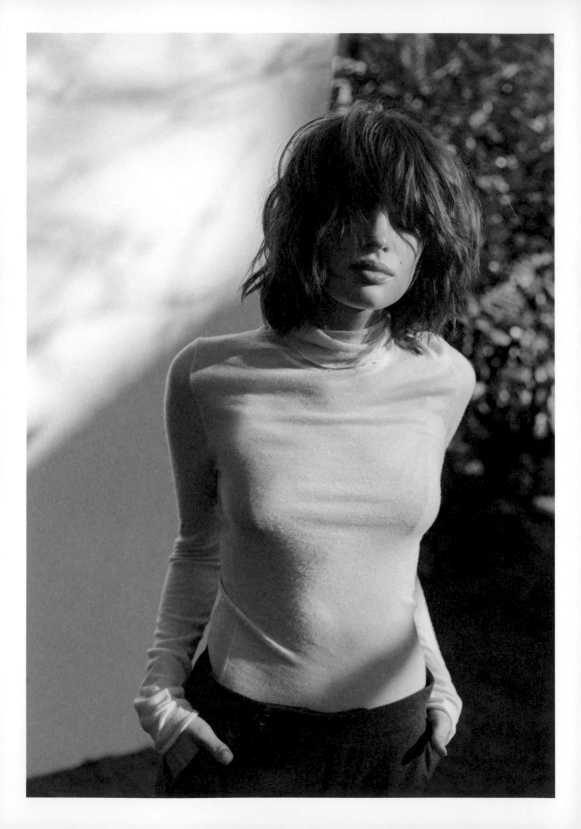

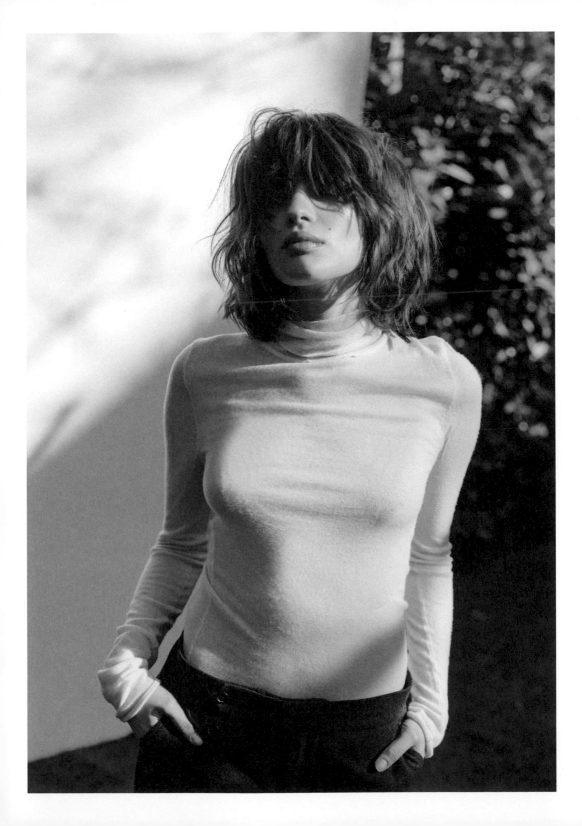

~~YOU CAN'T HAVE EVERYTHING~~

There's still a very rigid side of hairdressing that tells women they can't have a particular haircut because it doesn't suit them, or they can't colour their hair a particular colour because they can't carry it off. There's too much 'you can't have'. I believe that everyone can have everything (within reason). It's really about how things are adapted to suit you and your needs. Everyone can achieve whatever they want with their hair, one way or the other. You may just have to understand the downside or the constraints of doing something, but there's no reason why you can't do what you want. If you want to take your hair from black to white-blonde, you can. There's nothing stopping you – you just need to be aware that it will take a number of appointments to get there and there will be damage. Don't let anyone tell you no.

~~YOU HAVE TO CUT YOUR HAIR EVERY SIX WEEKS~~

This makes me laugh. We are not in the eighties any more; women really don't have those very structural high-maintenance styles that need excessive and regular pruning. This rule may have applied when haircuts were very precise and graphic but now – thanks to colour techniques like balayage and how we're cutting hair – you can actually enjoy the growing-out process. Unless you have a short or very specific length that you want to maintain then do not feel pressured into getting a trim every six weeks.

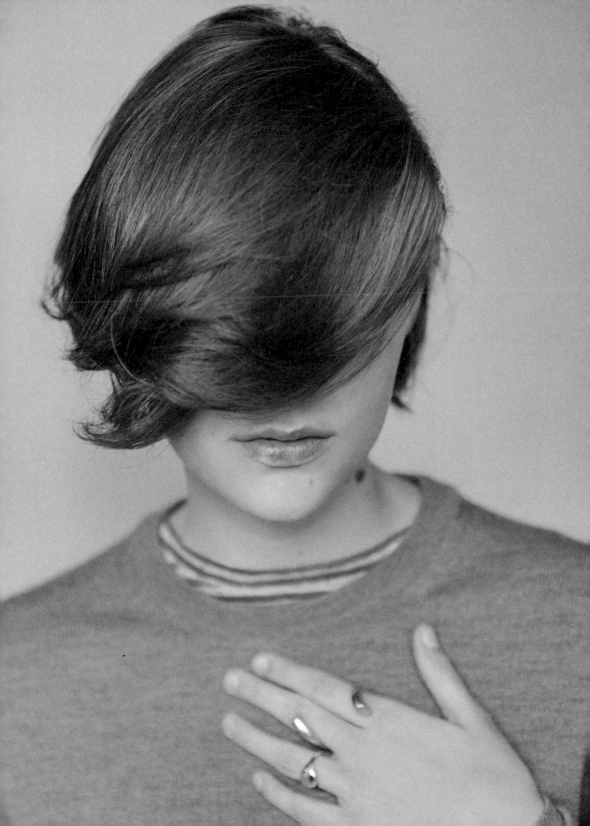

RULES WORTH FOLLOWING

As much as I take great pleasure in ignoring what I am told I *should* do, there are a handful of guidelines that have never steered me off course.

NEVER PUT HEAT DIRECTLY ONTO WET HAIR

If you value healthy hair this is one rule you should never ignore. If you place a heated styling tool – such as a straightening iron or a curling tong – directly onto wet hair you will quickly (almost instantly) boil the hair residing in the hair shaft. This then blisters the hair and irrevocably damages the protective cuticle layer, meaning that your hair will become frizzy, broken and weak, and almost impossible to style. No amount of repairing masks can fix this kind of damage – the only way to be rid of it is to cut your hair.

NEVER CUT YOUR HAIR YOURSELF

This is a rule for so many reasons. Perhaps the two most important ones are these:

1) A hairdresser has been trained to cut hair and they instinctively know things like where you'd benefit from some layers, what you need to frame your face and the right implement (whether that be scissors or a razor) to create soft and flattering ends.

2) Much of a hairdresser's value lies in their experience and opinion. They will perhaps suggest something new, or a tweak, that you might not have thought of before. Essentially, if you cut your hair yourself you are limiting your options and perhaps not achieving your hair's full potential.

There are, of course, exceptions to the rule and if you are extremely talented with a pair of scissors and you have exquisite taste then go for it. I have seen a couple of models cut their own hair (and do it very well) so there are some people who can pull it off but they are most definitely few.

ALWAYS CHECK OUT A HAIRDRESSER'S WORK BEFORE MAKING AN APPOINTMENT

Any decent hairdresser in this day and age should have an Instagram account where they share examples of their work and what inspires them. If they don't, you have to ask yourself what they are trying to hide. Your hair is such an integral part of your whole look and you must be confident that you're placing its fate in the hands of someone who shares your sense of what is good taste and who will deliver what you want.

DON'T BOTHER WITH ROLLERS

If I could start a campaign to ban rollers I would. I think they create a very old-fashioned style that immediately ages you. The *only* time they are appropriate is if you are deliberately creating a retro, Veronica Lake look with cascading waves. Whatever you think you need rollers for, trust me, there is a better way to achieve it. If you want more volume you can easily achieve that with just your hands and your hairdryer (see Your Hair Routine) and if you want to create a wave, a curling tong or wand will give you a far more modern shape.

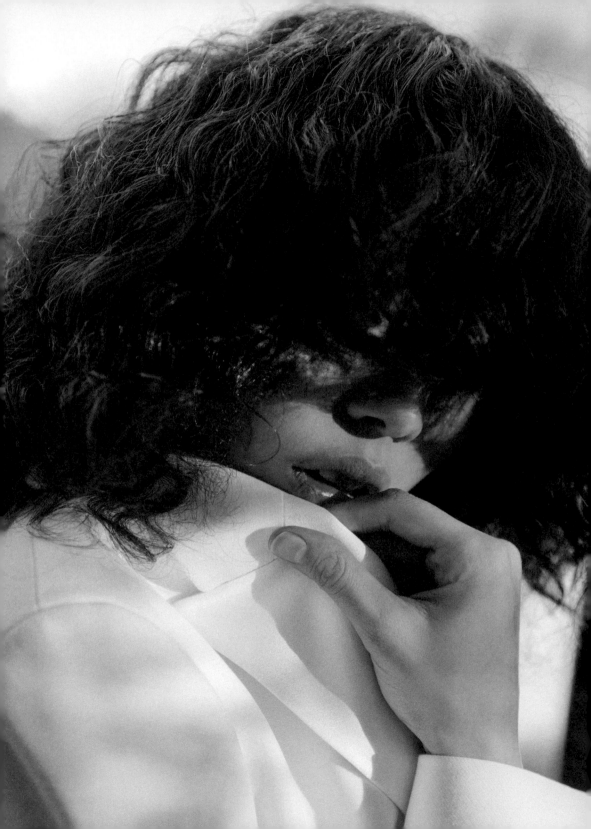

HAIR

AT

ALL

AGES

'We're about great hair at any age'

Hershesons is emphatically not about young hair – we're about great hair at *any* age – and I can wholeheartedly say that there is no reason whatsoever that great hair should be the preserve of the young. There is no such thing as 'age appropriate' hair. Getting older means something very different to women now than it once did. Perhaps a couple of decades ago, women of a certain age cut their hair and had a lilac rinse. Now they recognise no such limitations. The beauty industry has finally caught up with this new ageless mentality with respected beauty bible *Allure* magazine even going so far as to ban the words 'anti-ageing' from their pages.

Eternally chic older icons, including Dame Helen Mirren, former US First Lady Michelle Obama, model Maye Musk, and actresses Diane Keaton and Jane Fonda, all serve as bold inspiration for women who look forward to ageing beautifully. And you only have to look at the likes of Jennifer Aniston, Sofia Vergara, Julianne Moore and Aishwarya Rai to see the suggestion that women over the age of forty should cut their hair for what it is: utter bullshit.

Having said that, while our attitude to ageing has been turned on its head, there is no denying that hair will look and behave differently at different points of your life, and the older you get the more challenges you will be presented with. I like to think of it as my job to equip you properly so that you can meet these challenges head on and triumph.

THE TEEN YEARS

Studies show that our hair is at its best when we are between the ages of twelve and fourteen, before colouring, perming and heat styling begins to take its toll. Most teenagers are enjoying the best hair they are ever likely to have but – though it's rare – some teenage girls can experience hair loss thanks to their ever fluctuating hormones. This thinning occurs when the hormone testosterone converts into DHT (dihydrotestosterone) and shrinks the hair follicles, causing the hair to fall out. Occasionally medicines, such as the pill, are behind this hormonal imbalance but a doctor or health practitioner should be able to say for sure.

By far the most common complaint amongst teenage girls when it comes to their hair is grease. Rapid hormonal changes associated with the onset of puberty can result in excess sebum, which, as we know, can lead to acne breakouts on the face, chest and back. It's a similar situation on the scalp. Too much oil makes hair appear lank and greasy, while the excess sebum can block follicles and irritate the scalp, resulting in embarrassing dandruff.

Clarifying shampoos designed for a flaky scalp – such as those by Kérastase, Oribe and Phyto – will help to remove superfluous oils and calm inflammation, while soothing and balancing masks and tonics should help to bring the scalp back in line. Dry shampoo is invaluable – it will absorb excess oils from the scalp and roots and refresh hair as the day wears on – but do not allow the powder to build up on the scalp or this could lead to more inflammation.

The teen years are prime time to play with your hairstyle and colour – before you may be limited by what employers consider acceptable. If you experiment with bleach and crazy colours, just remember that while your hair is probably the strongest it's likely ever to be it is not immune to damage. Counter any experimentation with strengthening shampoos, conditioners and intensive treatments.

The teen cheat sheet
· Speak to your GP if you are losing hair and you're taking the pill.
· Don't let a greasy scalp let you down. Invest in Kérastase Bain Divalent, which regulates the excess sebum resulting in oily hair.
· Dry shampoo is brilliant but do not allow the product to build up on your scalp otherwise this could lead to sensitivity, redness and flakes.
· Wash your hair regularly – around every other day – to remove product build-up and excess oils. Do not be tempted to wash it more frequently than that or you may strip your scalp of moisture and encourage it to produce even more sebum.

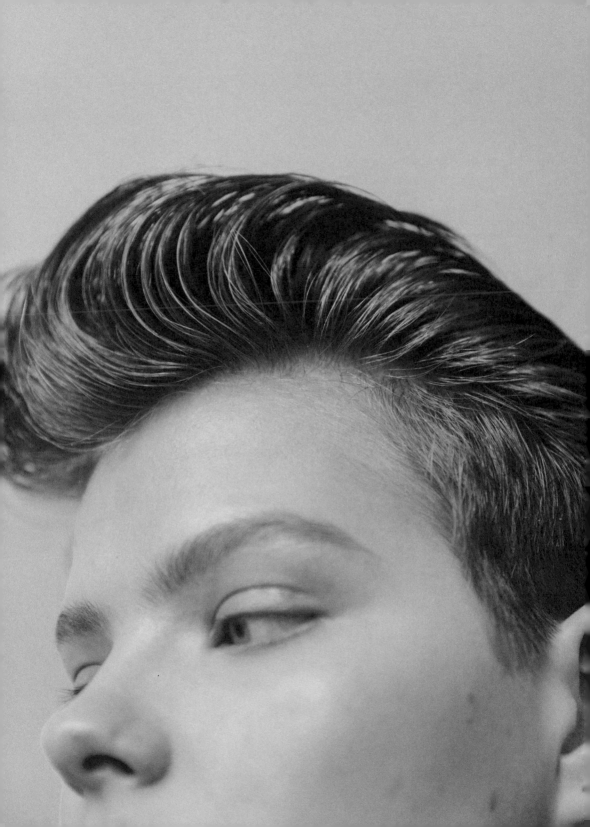

MOTHERHOOD

There is no such thing as a textbook pregnancy and one woman's experience might be the complete opposite of someone else's. Generally speaking though, your hair goes through some kind of miraculous transformation when you're expecting. The hormones that your body produces while it is growing a baby can result in changes in hair growth and texture, and most of the time it's for the good. Your hair may very well grow faster and fall out less, which will produce a pretty impressive head of hair. (The downside to this though is that you may see more hair elsewhere on your body too.) Your hair shouldn't require too much maintenance while you're pregnant, simply because it will be doing a great job of looking after itself.

There has been much debate over the years about whether it's safe to dye your hair during this time. The general medical consensus is that the chemicals in permanent and semi-permanent hair colours are not considered to be highly toxic and therefore are safe to use when pregnant and even when breastfeeding. Many women err on the side of caution and opt not to dye their hair during the first twelve weeks of pregnancy.

Postpartum hair loss is quite common and absolutely nothing to worry about. Most new mothers will see some hair loss around the third month after birth though this may be delayed if you're breastfeeding. It's understandable that you may be alarmed initially but it's just your hormone levels and your rate of hair growth and shedding returning to pre-pregnancy normality. If someone could bottle the hair-boosting effects of pregnancy they would be a very wealthy person indeed.

Five-minute hair for the mum on the run
· Work a little styling cream through dry hair with your hands to tame any frizz and flyaways.
· Twist your hair up into what I call a 'mum bun', which is really just a topknot. Gather your hair into a pony on the top of your head and twist the length of your hair around itself.
· Secure with a Syd Pin. What makes this pin so brilliant is that with a little practice you can secure your bun in place using only one hand. That's good news when your other hand is busy with a baby.

AGE IS JUST A NUMBER

Various studies show that women are more concerned with their hair thinning than they are any other age-related change in their appearance. I can completely understand why. The odd line and wrinkle adds character to your face; laughter lines, for example, suggest that you're a happy person and enjoy a laugh. But thinning hair doesn't add anything to your character; in fact, it can do quite the opposite and make you feel like shit.

In reality women start to lose a little hair density from around the age of twenty, though they might not notice it until forty or so. Sebum production starts to take a nosedive, which results in dry and unruly hair. Essentially, with age hair becomes thinner, drier and less elastic, and the diameter of each individual strand can decrease until the follicle stops producing hair altogether. Oestrogen levels begin to drop off with the onset of menopause, and androgens – or male hormones – can climb, which can lead to further thinning on the top and at the front of the scalp. Sorry to be the bearer of bad news.

There is news to get majorly excited about, though. The big beauty brands who traditionally have spent staggeringly huge sums of money on skincare research and development at the expense of haircare, are now redirecting their cash. It has come to light over the last few years that a lot of the powerful active ingredients in skincare can actually have a big benefit to hair too. This is why the 'care' category is looking better than ever, and you can really expect great results from your haircare products. Look for shampoos, masks and intensive treatments containing panthenol, niacinamide (also known as vitamin B3) and caffeine, which have been shown to penetrate hair follicles and increase hair diameter. The increase is only a matter of microns but when that is seen over the entire head it can make a huge difference.

Minoxidil is currently the only FDA-approved treatment for hair growth (other supplements can contribute to your overall health and so make you less likely to lose hair). You can find it in Regaine or Rogaine depending on where you are in the world. Though it's important to note that it doesn't work for everyone and if you *do* see an improvement with it, your hair will go back to normal if you stop using it. But remember, not all hair loss is

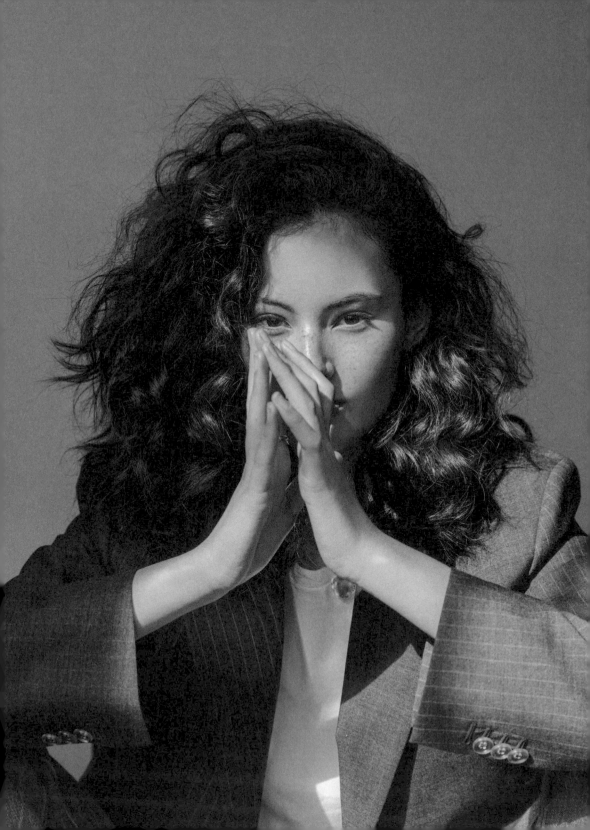

down to ageing. If it coincides with acne and/or increased facial and body hair then you should see your doctor or health practitioner to get to the bottom of it.

As for your style; it's easy to get weighed down with a 'signature' hairstyle as you get older but, in my opinion, you should embrace the changes your hair is going through and change up your style too. Dame Helen Mirren is a fabulous example of someone who doesn't allow her age to influence her styling choices. I have had the privilege to work with her on a few occasions, even once on a cover for *Allure* magazine, and I am in awe of her eagerness to experiment; her bright pastel-pink dye job (inspired by *America's Next Top Model*) that she debuted at the BAFTAs a few years back remains a favourite.

If your hairdresser asks your age, then chances are they are cutting your hair with some preconceived idea of what 'older' women should look like and that usually translates into something short and generic-looking. If that's the case, perhaps now is a good time to change your stylist too. No doubt your style has changed over the years, your fashion tastes will have evolved, the way you wear your make-up is likely different too, and it makes sense that your hair is part of this gradual transformation. But, more important than all of this, is how your hair makes you *feel*; if it's not helping you to feel confident and you don't feel that it accurately represents your personality then it is time for a change.

GREYING GRACEFULLY

Never before has grey hair been so wonderfully celebrated as it is right now; it's on the catwalk, on TV and in our magazines and newspapers. More women than ever are making the bold decision to stop dyeing altogether and embrace grey, and the results couldn't be more beautiful. It's testament to great influential grey-haired women, including models Kristen McMenamy and Maye Musk, British *Vogue*'s Sarah Harris, and Christine Lagarde, who is the director of the International Monetary Fund, that women who don't even have any grey hairs yet are faking the shade with dye.

I don't know if we'll really understand why hair goes grey for some time yet but it's not unusual for most women to have a few renegade strands by the time they're thirty (or even younger as the case can be). By the time women reach the age of fifty, usually around half their hair will be grey. Contrary to what most people think, grey hair isn't actually a colour, it is in fact a combination of normal pigmented hair and hair that has lost its pigment entirely making it appear white. If you have an entire head of grey this means that you have lost the pigment from every single strand of hair. People often think that dark-haired women turn grey earlier than their fairer counterparts; actually this is just down to the white strands being more noticeable against darker hair than against paler. Also, you can forget the old wives' tale that if you pluck out a grey hair two more will grow in its place – it's nonsense.

The age that you'll turn grey is a tricky thing to predict but genetics play a huge role in its onset – if either of your parents went grey at an early age it's safe to assume that you will too. Hormones, illness, stress, and physical and emotional traumas have also been linked to going grey early.

If you don't like your newly grey hair there's not really much you can do about it; and although occasionally the rumour-mill goes into overdrive with speculation that some major brand or other is about to launch the antidote to greying, such a product has yet to materialise. Other studies suggest that taking large doses of certain B vitamins can start the reversal process but there is much more research needed before we'll know for certain. Until then we'll have to make do with the magic that is hair dye.

It's a common misconception that hair becomes coarse as it goes grey; actually, it's most likely to become thinner and drier because it's proba-ble that you'll also be producing less sebum than before. Look after your grey hair much in the same way as you did before; you can colour it and perm it just as you once did. Perms and smoking can occasionally turn grey hair slightly yellow but this can be corrected with blue- and purple-based shampoos, which will neutralise the brassiness.

If you're ready to put down the dye and embrace your new colouring I suggest waiting until all of your hair is grey in tone. Even with the best intentions, patches of grey here and there is never a good look in my book. Maintain your bottled colour until you're ready for the big reveal.

HEALTH

The state of your health and even the medications and treatments that you might be on will be having some effect on the condition of your hair. For example, some drugs used to attack cancer cells can attack your hair follicles too. Chances are this is something you either have first- or second-hand knowledge of as there are not many of us who remain untouched by cancer in some way or another. Unfortunately, while undoubtedly traumatic in its own right, there is nothing you can do to completely protect your hair against the aggression of chemotherapy; the very thing that makes chemotherapy effective at destroying rapidly dividing cancerous cells also makes it devastating to the hair on your head, your pubic area and your eyebrows and lashes. Hair loss usually occurs around two weeks after that initial round of chemotherapy but often it's not noticeable to others until 50 per cent of the hair has been lost. Once you have seen your treatment to its end your hair growth will slowly return to normal though you may see quite drastic changes in its texture and structure, and it's not uncommon to have straight or wavy hair naturally, only to have a surprising flood of curls after your hair begins to grow back.

It can be emotionally traumatising to anyone undergoing treatment but it's particularly so for women as so much of a woman's self-expression and personality are bound up with her hair. Everyone faces and tackles this challenge differently. Some women choose to wear a Cold Cap or use a cooling system while undergoing treatment, to cool the scalp in an effort to reduce the trauma to the hair. In some patients it can slow the rate of hair loss but it doesn't work for everyone and can be quite uncomfortable to wear.

Another option is to take matters into your own hands and shave it off yourself, either when the thinning has become noticeable or – as is the case with some women – before you have even started treatment. This course of action is obviously not for everyone and it can, for some, add more stress to an already traumatic event but others find it empowering to take decisive action. There are even charities who will collect the shorn hair and use it to create wigs for others going through a similar situation.

Wigs are a fantastic option to see you through. The hairdresser Trevor Sorbie founded a charity called My New Hair (mynewhair.org), which supports and trains stylists and salons to provide a styling service for people looking for a wig due to cancer and medical hair loss. Their website is also a great resource for advice and guidance on choosing a wig and finding the right stylist.

But regardless of how you choose to tackle your hair loss it's important to know that you are supported, and however crap this all feels right now in the moment, some day you'll be on the other side of it. Many oncology centres work with charities who want to spend time with you, help you with any decisions you have to make and, hopefully, make the ordeal that little bit less stressful. Whether you need some styling tips for your wig, want to know how to draw in some convincing-looking brows or how to apply false eyelashes, there are people and resources out there just waiting to meet you. Ask your consultant to point you in the right direction and if you're in the UK check out LookGoodFeelBetter.co.uk – an exceptional organisation, which, with the help of volunteers, helps you look and feel your best when you're going through a shitty time.

Some things worth considering if you decide to wear a wig:

Colour: Chemotherapy can temporarily alter your skin tone so you shouldn't necessarily choose a wig that's identical to your natural hair colour. Look at shades a touch lighter than your original hair colour or see this as an opportunity to experiment with shades.

Take a picture of yourself before you start your treatment so that your hairstylist – or whoever you buy your wig from – can see what you looked like prior to thinning.

Synthetic wigs tend to be cheaper than those made of real hair. They maintain their style for longer and need less maintenance but you can't use heated styling tools on them or you risk melting the strands.

Wigs made from real hair can look more natural, and can be styled in the same way you would your own hair, but they will need regular styling and washing. If you're opting for a real hair wig try and buy one with more length than you need so that you can have it cut and styled yourself.

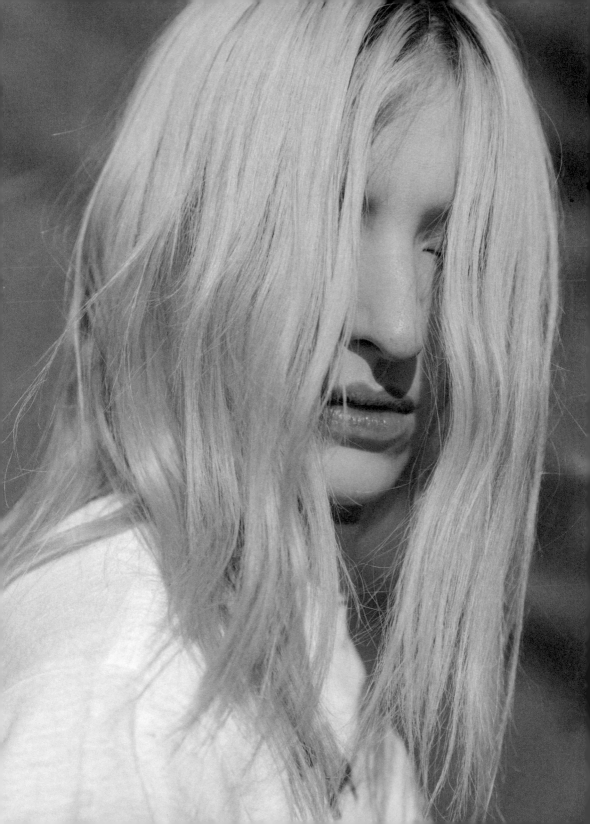

Avoid wigs that are lined with anything irritating, itchy or uncomfortable, otherwise it will drive you to distraction. It's also important that it is well ventilated so your scalp doesn't become unbearably hot. Many wigs are designed for women who already have some hair so it's not a given that all of them will be comfortable to wear on bare skin. A thin, soft mesh base where the strands have been sewn in by hand tends to be the most comfortable of the lot.

Wearing a cap underneath or anchoring your wig in place with something called a Wig Hugger (a gel-like band) or body tape will minimise the chances of it slipping around when your scalp becomes sweaty.

THYROID ISSUES

It is believed that women are five to eight times more likely to experience thyroid problems than men. This is usually hyperthyroidism (an overactive thyroid) and hypothyroidism (an underactive thyroid). The thyroid is a butterfly-shaped gland nestled in the lower neck that produces hormones. There are a whole host of symptoms that go hand in hand with a misbehaving thyroid – from weight loss or gain, fatigue, muscle cramping and insomnia, depending on whether your thyroid is under- or over-performing.

However, both conditions can result in massive changes to your hair. An overactive thyroid can cause thinning and excess shedding while an underactive thyroid results in dry and brittle hair with obvious signs of thinning (this doesn't just affect the hair on your head so you may notice changes in your body and pubic hair too).

Unlike other types of hair loss that confine themselves to the hairline or the front of the scalp, this kind of hair loss is far more uniform and impacts the whole scalp so you're unlikely to even notice you're thinning until you have already lost a fair bit of hair.

Thankfully, a full course of treatment for your thyroid should rectify most of these issues so your hair can get back to its former lustrous self. Either way, you must see your GP or health practitioner if you're in any way concerned about your thyroid; they'll do a full blood work to get to the bottom of things.

Whether it's a flu or something more serious, as a 'non-essential' element your hair is usually the first thing to look a little the worse for wear when you're ill. When you can find the energy – or indeed the enthusiasm – once again try the following to perk yourself up:

Use a scalp mask such as Philip Kingsley Exfoliating Scalp Mask. If your hair has been left unwashed for a little while it will have likely built up dirt, product and bacteria on your scalp. Dampen your hair and apply the mask directly to your scalp, give it a little massage and allow it to do its thing for ten to twenty minutes before rinsing it out.

Strengthen fragile post-poorly hair. Davines Natura Tech Energizing Gel is like a shot of espresso for your scalp. Apply it in a grid directly to your scalp after you have washed your hair and use your fingertips to distribute it. It's satisfyingly cool and tingly.

Apply a nourishing and gorgeously cocooning hair mask, it's just as relaxing and luxurious as a face mask. Carve half an hour out of your day to wallow in a hot bath and indulge in a strengthening and rehydrating mask such as Phyto Phytokératine Extrême Exceptional Mask.

Book yourself in for a blow dry. When you have been feeling under the weather there is nothing like allowing someone else to pamper you to make you feel like yourself again. Book into a salon that you love the look of and enjoy allowing someone else to wash, dry and style your hair for a change.

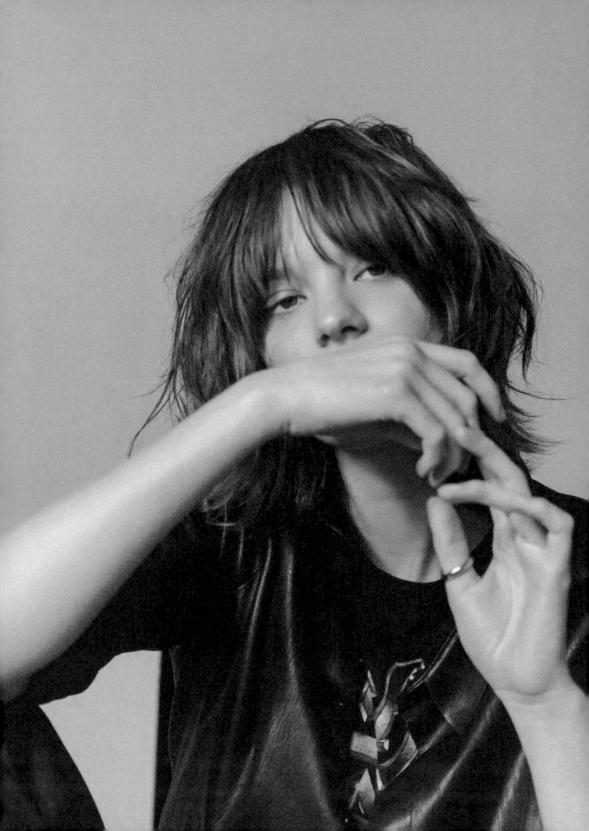

HAIR
GOALS

'Chopping off
your hair can
be liberating
and confidence
boosting'

Despite what some hairdressers would have you believe, hair is not hard. Besides, more often than not the most lusted-after looks are those that look relaxed and effortless.

You should never feel intimidated by a hairstyle or worry that it is not *you*. Who is to say that something won't look good on you? Give something a try and see for yourself. At the end of the day, it is only hair and if you don't like a hairstyle you can wash it out and start again, and if you don't like a cut, guess what – it will grow back. That's the wonderful thing about hair; it renews itself, nothing is ever permanent, so you can afford to be a little experimental on occasion.

I have been in this business for some time now and I can tell you there are some styles that resurface time and time again, that are always popular with our clients and are eternally covetable. They also happen to be the kinds of styles that you might assume are tricky to nail down. Well, they're not and I'm going to tell you exactly how you can get a piece of the action.

COOL-GIRL WAVES

Bedhead hair, surfer-girl waves, Californian waves, rock-chic hair, whatever you want to call them, these loose, undone relaxed waves are at the top of everyone's wish list.

It might surprise you to know that these 'effortless' waves actually require a little effort and some forward planning. It all begins with the right cut. Ask your hairdresser for some invisible layers here and there. Unlike traditional layers, these are cut into the underneath of the hair and changing up the length in this way will encourage a wave and allow you to tong your hair easily. As hard as you might try, you cannot create these kinds of mussed-up waves on hair that is all one length; you won't end up with the separation you're looking for and instead you will get a much blockier, more retro wave.

Next up, colour. Ask your colourist to add some depth to your hair; maybe make the roots a bit darker, the mid-lengths and ends a bit lighter and a slight variation in shade throughout, so that when you add your wave your hair looks more beachy. A solid, all-over colour works when your hair is styled straight but when you are encouraging movement, shape and separation, adding multiple shades of the same colour will enhance the 'undone' finish.

A tong with a barrel that's just the right size is essential when creating this look. You want a medium-sized barrel about 2.5 centimetres in diameter. Our Tourmaline Professional Curling Tong is perfect for the job. Forget about combing and precisely sectioning your hair and pinning it out of the way; this is a nonchalant, lazy wave so any kind of uniformity is unwelcome. Eventually with a bit of practice this step will become intuitive but until then aim for sections a couple of inches wide. If your sections are too small – say half a centimetre or a centimetre – then you'll end up with a much more defined, tighter curl. If your sections are too big then you run the risk of creating weak waves that drop out almost instantly. You're aiming for a happy medium between the two.

Now, the tonging. First of all you must prep your hair with a heat-protection product to minimise damage. Start on top of your head – the outer layers of hair – as this is what people see the most. No one sees the underneath of your hair so you don't need much of a wave there. Leave a couple of centimetres of the roots and the ends out of the tong and twist the section of hair between your thumb and forefinger as you feed it around the barrel. Leaving the roots and ends slightly straighter will create a more modern and cool wave.

Work from front to back and pull each section of hair over your shoulder and round to the front of your face and don't worry if you don't get to every single section. Remember, uniformity is the enemy. Hold the hair around the tong for a few seconds as the curl develops and remember to hold the ends out. Which direction you tong your hair isn't so important; towards your face, away from your face, it really doesn't matter so do whatever feels most comfortable. One thing is necessary, though; make sure your tong is always facing downwards with the cable end facing up towards the ceiling when you're tonging the front sections; this will ensure the right-shaped wave. The tong should be quite horizontal to your head when you're doing the rest. Remove the tong from your hair, hold the curl in your hand a second or two while it cools and then use your fingers to bring some separation to the wave.

Tonging the front sections of hair so that they properly frame your face can be a little tricky. Here's my tip: when you have tonged the front sections, quickly tuck them behind your ears before they have had a chance to cool. In this way you are basically using your ears as styling tools. Once the sections have cooled, free them from behind your ears and loosen up the texture with your fingers to frame your face.

I suggest that until you are comfortable tonging and it starts to feel like second nature, don't use a mirror, but do everything by feel alone. This may sound counterintuitive but, trust me, learning this technique while looking in the mirror presents some challenges. The mirror, obviously, shows you everything in reverse so your brain is telling you to go one way and the mirror is telling you to go in the other. It's unnecessarily confusing and I'm willing to bet you can do a fine job without it.

Sometimes hair can appear *too* tonged, which is a very contrived look. If that's the case just take a pair of straightening irons and lightly tap at intervals down the length of the curl. It will loosen the shape and make it look more relaxed and less prom-like.

Don't be afraid to get your hands in your hair and shake it around. It takes some confidence to painstakingly tong your hair only to roughly manhandle it but you have got to be prepared to destroy it a little. Work some Almost Everything Cream through the lengths and rub sections between your fingertips to create that sexy slept-in texture. Finish with a mist of hairspray and you're done.

RETURN OF THE CUT

We are living in the age of the haircut. Chopping off your hair can be liberating and sexy and confidence boosting. As a hairdresser I can tell you that it is a huge honour when a woman entrusts you with her hair, when she's willing to let you cut away her longer lengths. So much of a woman's comfort and feeling of stability lies in her long hair and to give permission to someone to cut that away is a big deal. I have to give a shout out to a handful of brilliant beauty journalists who have at one point or another given me free rein with my scissors and allowed me to take their hair shorter: Alessandra Steinherr, Sali Hughes and Joanna McGarry. Hairdressers, of course, are loving this turn of events as it allows us to do what we enjoy most – cut. LA-based Jen Atkin is really championing shorter hair and is responsible for cuts seen on Kendall Jenner, Khloé Kardashian and Jenna Dewan Tatum.

When I started, models could only have long hair, and if their hair was short they just wouldn't get booked for shows or campaigns. But now you just have to look at any fashion show to see that it's all about individuality and unique looks, and nowadays a bolder cut can really elevate a model and get them even more work. Bella Hadid and Kendall Jenner spring to mind as two who have added to their uniqueness with a shorter style.

It's not necessarily about a length – as you'll see below – it's way more about the shape. So whether your hair is skimming your shoulder, or peeking out just below your ears, it's making a statement for sure. Here's my round-up of what I consider to be the best – and most loved – shorter looks right now.

BOB

It has taken a while for the traditional bob to come back around again but if Bella Hadid's glossy do is anything to go by it's back for good. Bella's chin-grazing cut is everything a bob should be; it's both playful and edgy and looks just as show-stopping with a fringe and without. But a bob doesn't necessarily have to be worn neat; it can look dishevelled and cool as I have demonstrated with cuts for Victoria Beckham and Sienna Miller. A bob is a very specific length so be prepared to get very regular trims.

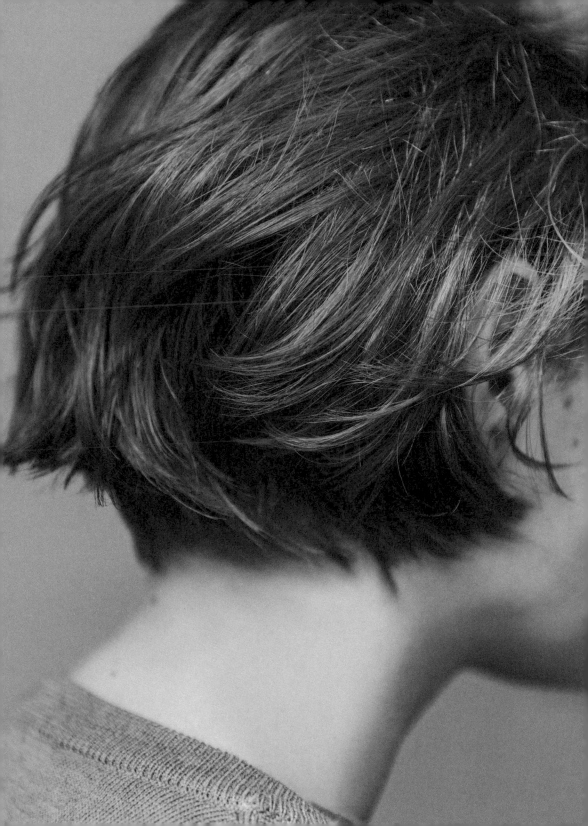

ANTIBOB

A traditional bob cut involves heavy corners and precision down to every single hair – it's very rock 'n' roll. The Antibob, in comparison, ignores those rules and instead is based on a reverse triangle shape that meets at the lowest point at the back of the head. The result is a style that's longer at the back and shorter at the front. It looks a little DIY, but deliberately so, and it looks more nonchalant and relaxed than a traditional bob.

SHAG

There are those who probably thought the seventies shag would never see the light of day again, but thankfully they were wrong. The difference between the shag of today and the look that was made popular a few decades ago, is that today's incarnation is more relaxed, a little longer and looks incredible with a fringe. A shag cut has a few layers of varying lengths and – as demonstrated by Bella Freud, Kate Moss, Sienna Miller, Emmanuel Alt, and models Freja Beha Erichsen and Edie Campbell – looks very cool.

BAD BOB

This is something I created for Sienna Miller a few years back for a film. We had been planning it for years but originally we were going to take it even shorter, more along the lines of Winona Ryder's hair in the nineties. Instead we came up with what I call a Bad Bob – I mean, it looks great but technically it's the things you're not meant to do with a bob. It has a bit of a Parisian feel, with torn ends, and it's certainly a bit more boyish and tougher than longer hair. At its heart, and from the front, it's a regular bob, but if you were to look around the back you'd find an undercut, which really gives the look some edge and adds another layer of interest when the rest of the hair is put up into a bun.

MIDDY

There's something very polished and glamorous about perfect mid-length hair that skims the shoulder. Just think of Olivia Palermo and Emily Weiss. This is another look that requires regular trims to maintain that precise length; just a couple of centimetres longer and it can become dowdy.

GLOSSY NATURAL CURLS

It's really great to see women embracing their curls again; whether they are born with them or they're curls that they have created with a perm. However, at the risk of repeating myself, a good cut lies at the heart of a great head of curls – even if it's a perm. We know from experience gained from developing our own perming techniques in-salon that the end result is still entirely dependent on the way we cut the hair beforehand. Refer back to It All Starts with a Good Haircut if you need more guidance but essentially you're looking for a hairdresser who has skill and experience with cutting curls – sadly, that's not everyone. As for the cut, you need to ask for some clever layering, particularly around the front of your face, so that your curls are full of body and lie just so.

Curls do not – and should not – have to be crispy. The eighties were inspiring in many ways but the crispy, untouchable curls that have come to symbolise that decade can stay there. Avoiding these is easier than you might think – just don't go anywhere near a can of mousse.

When it comes to actually creating beautifully defined and touchable curls it's really all about the product that you apply to your hair while it is still wet rather than anything you apply afterwards as a finisher. This is when you add definition and reduce frizz.

Work a little styling cream through your hair with your fingers to distribute it evenly – our Almost Everything Cream really excels here.

Oils are also brilliant for curly hair as they rehydrate and give life to its shape. I love to use Kérastase Elixir Ultime, the original Moroccanoil or Phytoelixir Oil – they all essentially do the same thing. How much oil you need to use will really depend on the thickness of your hair. Until you are used to using it start with just a small pump and work it from roots to ends or just anywhere your hair feels particularly parched. Add more until you notice a difference in how your hair feels; when it feels moisturised it's time to stop.

Dig out the diffuser attachment to your hairdryer, flip your head upside down and allow your hair to pool in sections into the well of the diffuser. Don't be tempted to touch it or mess with it – you need to exercise some patience here. Allow the hair to cook a little in the diffuser until it is completely dry. Then you can release it. While it might not be new, this technique is tried and tested and guaranteed to produce bountiful defined curls without the frizz.

Unlike straighter hair – which, in my opinion, always looks best a day after washing – curly hair really comes to life when it is freshly shampooed so if you want the best curls of your life you really have to commit the time to wash them regularly.

FRINGES

Trends, by nature, come and go but the fringe is here to stay. Whether it's tousled or peek-a-boo, the fringe has always been – and will always be – utterly chic as proven by time-honoured fringe icons Jane Birkin, Brigitte Bardot, Marianne Faithfull and Julie Christie. Sienna Miller really represents, what I would call, modern-day fringe goals and in fact when clients bring inspiration pictures into the salon in order to have one cut in, it is more often than not a picture of Sienna with her signature seventies grown-out fringe.

Fringes come in many shapes and sizes; from the Side Sweep, which is really only halfway to a fringe and very easy to maintain, to the Blunt Chop, which is daring, graphic and requires 100 per cent commitment to its upkeep.

However, the most popular of them all is the Curtain Fringe, which has a seventies feel and is characterised by an eye-skimming length that's shorter in the middle, longer at the sides, and parted in the middle like, well, a curtain. It's exactly the kind of fringe Sienna and Georgia May Jagger are known for. The Curtain Fringe is in fact so popular that in 2017 Pinterest reported that searches for this style were up by 600 per cent. Women are clearly still obsessed with it.

So why is this style of fringe in particular so popular? It's flattering on almost everyone and on a scale of one to ten (one being so easy to maintain that you could do it in your sleep and ten being an absolute needy nightmare that requires you to dedicate a large chunk of your day to styling the thing) it's an easy four. It doesn't need to be perfectly straight – actually, it looks better when it isn't – it requires very little styling knowhow, looks great with both short and long hair, and hair that's worn up and down, and it grows out well. I like to think of this kind of fringe as an investment fringe because it looks great as it grows. What's not to like?

Take pictures of your favourite Curtain Fringe in to your hairdresser and ask them to adapt it for your features. Styling it at home couldn't be easier either. Apply the tiniest amount of styling cream to it while it is still wet and dry it with your hairdryer in different directions – alternating from side to side and away from your face – to create volume and shape.

Keeping a can of dry shampoo within reach is a good idea so you can refresh your fringe throughout the day (this is especially handy if you have oily skin as this can quickly make your fringe limp) and because there is less of it, it will likely need washing more often than the rest of your hair so be prepared to wash it – or at least dampen it – and dry it most mornings.

Fringe-drying tip: The best way to get your fringe to lie how you want it to is to wet it a bit and then aim your dryer at it (without a nozzle), ensuring that your dryer is parallel to the length of your hair. Keep your hairdryer further away from your hair than you normally would (but still close enough to dry) and then place a round brush underneath your fringe. Here's the really important bit; do not clamp your hand over your hair and the brush and do not use any kind of tension on the hair. If you use the brush to pull on the hair you will end up with a fringe that pings out in every direction and drives you mad. Instead just allow the hair to lie gently on top of the brush and roll the brush through it without pulling it. Dry your fringe this way and it will look awesome.

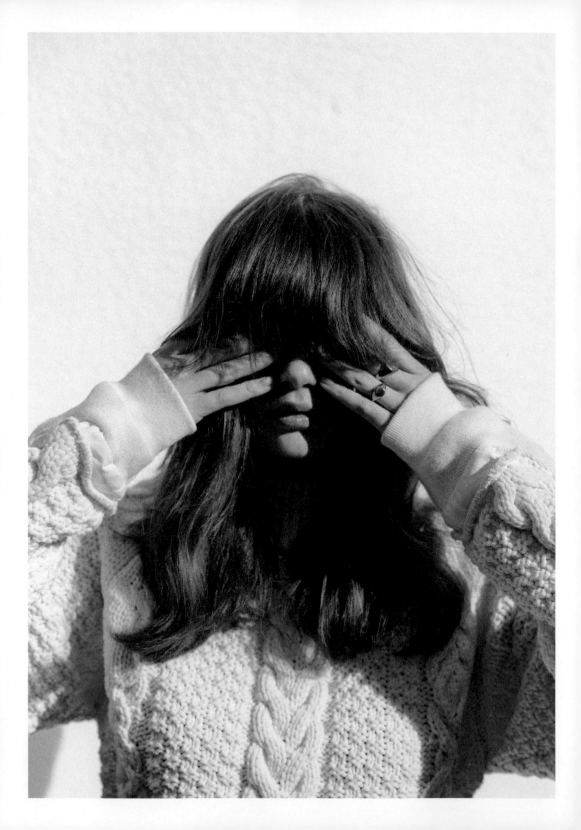

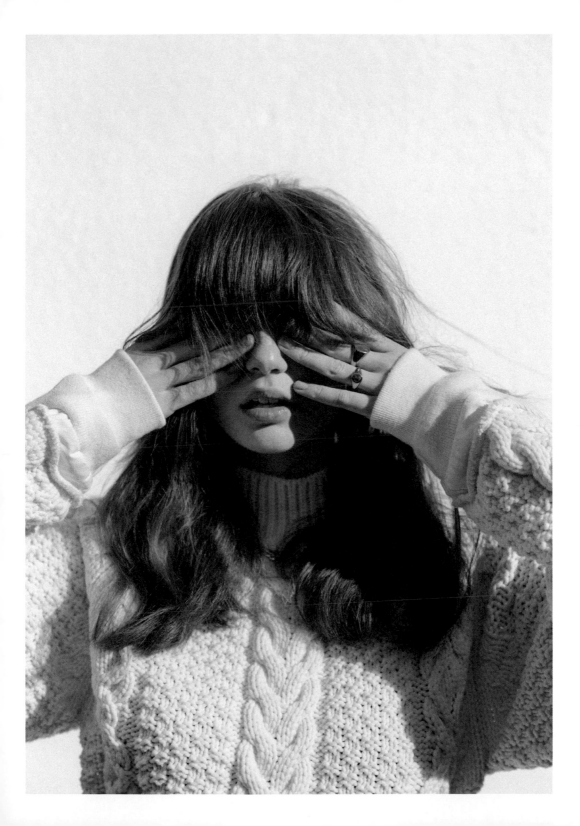

BRAIDING

Instagram, YouTube and Pinterest are awash with images and tutorials for braiding and it's a style that is guaranteed to turn up every season at the fashion shows and on every red carpet. Red-carpet regulars Jennifer Lawrence, Blake Lively, Gigi Hadid and Lupita Nyong'o understand the power of a statement braid on-camera and aside from their obvious beauty, a braid also serves a very useful purpose when it comes to dealing with day 2, or day 3 hair that is in need of a wash (this has 'festival' written all over it).

Braiding is a real art form and not something every stylist can do confidently. Some women seem to have a natural talent for braiding their own hair and those women have typically been braiding their hair – and their friends' – since they were young girls. If your own braiding skills are negligible but you want to be more proficient at it, then YouTube is really your best friend. Like anything, the best way to learn is to watch and repeat; practise on your own and on anyone else who will let you, until you have the technique nailed.

There are, of course, many variations on a braid. Here are just a few:

Cornrows are known as 'protective braids' as they keep the ends of Afro hair tucked away. They are braided very, very close to the scalp and have been used for centuries upon centuries as a style for Afro hair.

The French Braid is formed of just three sections that come together at the crown and stretch down to the nape of the neck. It's a very classic, youthful and naive look.

The Dutch Braid is kind of like its French counterpart but in reverse.

A Fishtail Braid is constructed from finer sections of hair and certainly requires some nimble fingers. In my opinion, the Fishtail is the most bohemian of the lot.

A Waterfall Braid is kind of ethereal looking and used to accentuate hair that is worn down.

Boxer Braids are controversial and while they have resurfaced in the media a lot over the last few years after being seen on various members of the Kardashian/Jenner clan, they are, in fact, fundamentally cornrows and have been worn by women with Afro hair since for ever. But it is true that athletes (and yes, boxers) favour the style because it efficiently keeps their hair out of their face.

The list is endless and I could go on for days, but suffice it to say that there are many options, requiring different levels of dexterity, which increases your odds of finding one you like and one you can actually create.

Braids have been a feature of our blow dry bars since the beginning and the Dirty Ballerina – which adds some edge to a classic and neat ballerina-style topknot – and the Side Stitch – which consists of tight cornrows on one side of the head – are consistent favourites amongst our clients. If you head over to our website you'll even find some useful tutorials demonstrating how you can create a handful of braids.

Clip-in hair extensions are brilliant to add some thickness and length to your hair before braiding; taking the time to add in a few pieces of hair here and there will give you a far more substantial braid. If your hair is thin and only producing a measly braid I suggest working some styling cream through it beforehand. This will give some guts and substance to the hair so you get a thicker braid. I always think that a braid is at its best when it looks as though it has been slept in; you can cheat that texture with a little hairspray and using your fingertips to rough up the braid and destroy it a little.

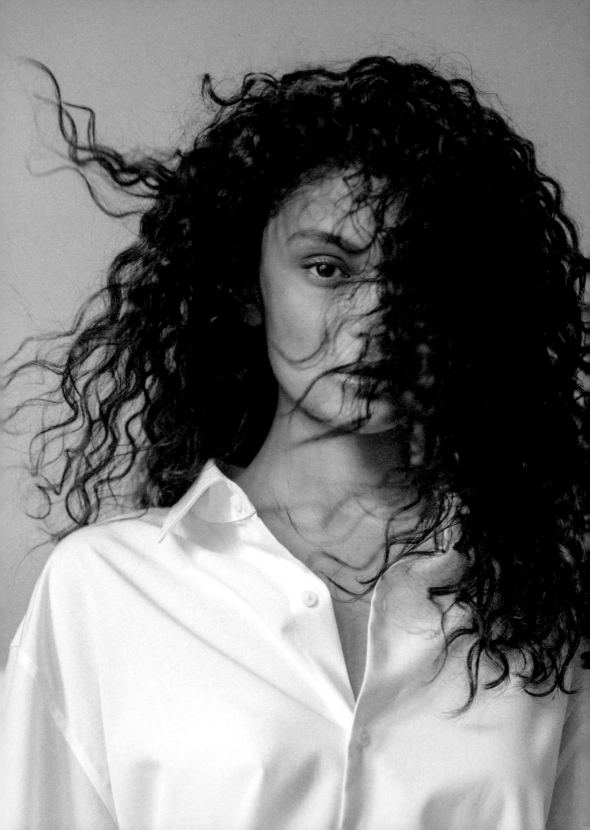

THE FLAVE

The 'Flave' is a relatively new styling technique that uses a straightening iron instead of a curling wand and emulates that kind of flat, graphic wave seen on the likes of Beyoncé and Khloé Kardashian. I think of it as the wave for women who don't want to look too 'done'. The Flave sits somewhere between nothing and something and gives you the merest 'hint' of movement, as though you have been rolling around in bed – it's about as far as you can get from 'LA tonged'. I came up with the technique when I was creating the look for Jonathan Saunders's SS15 show in London and despite how it looks, it could not be easier to achieve.

A straightening iron is the only tool that will give you this kind of kink so don't be tempted to try and create something similar with your curling wand because you will just be wasting your time. First, mist your hair with heat-protection spray (a must when using heated styling tools directly on your hair). Then feed your hair in sections through your straighteners, bending it from left to right as you go and clamping the straighteners down on your hair with each bend. This will create the kinks. It sounds fiddly but after five minutes it will feel quite natural and you'll pick up speed. Keep the roots out, as you would if you were tonging, and either use your fingers to muss up your hair once it has cooled or leave it as is if you want something more graphic.

THE PERM

A lot of women are scared of perms. Fact. I have put this down to the God-awful curly monstrosities we were subjected to in the eighties. Perms were mostly just all kinds of wrong then.

Trust me, the perms you knew then are dead and buried and the new and improved perm is a thing of beauty. The technology hasn't changed an awful lot – though there are some brands on the market now that are less damaging and contain no ammonia so they're a little kinder on hair – but the techniques used now are unrecognisable compared to what they once were.

We can now really gear a perm to do exactly what you want it to. Perming is – thankfully – no longer a case of simply coating the hair in perming solution and wrapping it around a rod. You can make your hair appear thicker, just by perming it. We have developed a technique at Hershesons (brought to life by our colourist Lily Bunting-Branch) called the 'Hair Thickening Perm' where we don't use rods or rollers; instead we plait the hair with the perming solution. This gives the softest, coolest wave (without being curly) and lots of body and volume.

If we want to create a very loose and relaxed curl, we'll set the hair around medium-sized foam pads instead of rollers. Of course the option is still there to use a roller or a rod if we're looking to end up with full and bouncy Julia Roberts-style curls. A perm should not look like a perm, it should look like naturally occurring beautiful curls.

Perms have always remained hugely popular in Asia – where hair tends to be naturally straight – while in the UK and the US you would count yourself lucky if you even found a salon that has a permer in residence. There was a time when every colourist knew how to perm but that's just no longer the case. Don't assume that your colourist can perm; the skills aren't necessarily transferrable. I consider perming to be a real art form and so much of the result is dependent on the skill of the technician.

You should care for your permed hair much in the same way as you would natural curls though it is vital that you don't allow your hair to get wet for at least forty-eight hours after having it permed; doing so could neutralise the solution and you'd lose your curls before you've even had a chance to enjoy them.

Perming *does* damage your hair to some extent, though the degree of damage really depends on what kind of condition your hair was in to begin with. Most likely there will be some damage and your hair will be left quite depleted of moisture. Choose your care products accordingly and use restorative and rehydrating masks containing keratin. Never use mousse to style your curls as this will instantly transport your look back to the eighties – which is everything we are trying to avoid – but instead use just a little oil or styling cream through your hair while it is still wet, and dry it using a diffuser to keep your curls looking their best.

STRAIGHTENING

I don't think there will ever be a time when women aren't having some kind of permanent straightening or smoothing treatment. Oddly, most of these treatments that come under the banner of 'straightening' don't actually straighten – most just smooth and remove frizz, which is really what most women want.

A Permanent, or Brazilian, Blow Dry uses a keratin solution to relax waves, smooth texture and soften frizz. Depending on the brand you may find that you can't wash your hair for a couple of days afterwards, or tie it up, so you should research the product on offer at your salon. Though it's called 'permanent' the results will soften slightly over the coming months and it will, of course, eventually grow out. It's brilliant for anyone with frizz because it softens the fluff without really altering the structure of the hair, and you're still left with plenty of movement and life in it. These treatments really do make life that little bit easier; your hair takes less time to style in the morning and it won't frizz up at the sight of humidity. The price really depends on where the salon is, with cities inevitably being more expensive, but you should expect to pay something around £250. There has been a real shift in the mindset of how women think about the Permanent Blow Dry. It's really seen now as a kind of hair hygiene, or maintenance, something to have done every three months or so to keep hair in check.

Yuko, or Japanese, straightening is a whole other board game. This treatment literally breaks down the bonds within the hair so that they can be 'reset' into a different shape – in this case, straight. It's much more expensive than a Permanent Blow Dry but the results won't fade, and you'll have straight hair until it grows out. Unlike a Permanent Blow Dry, Japanese straightening will leave behind no movement or texture so you're often left with poker, poker-straight hair.

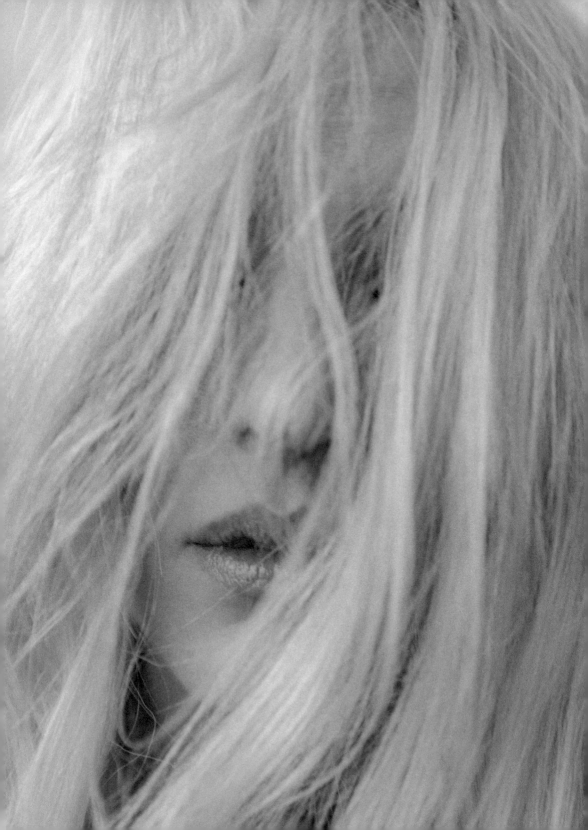

TAKE YOUR COLOUR TO THE NEXT LEVEL

'A great colourist
draws outside
the lines'

I truly believe that a lot of women get a colour without ever really knowing what's on offer. Most ask for an all-over colour, but I think they ask for that as a default because they do not know what other possibilities there are for them, except perhaps highlights. That's a failure on the part of the colourist. There are too many colourists to count in salons everywhere just doing what the client asks for without actually *looking* at their hair and offering their advice.

It is traditional for a salon to colour the hair first and then cut it, but at Hershesons we do it the other way around. It makes so much more sense to both us and the client for the colourists to come into the process once the cut is in place so they can paint *around* the haircut and bring out the bits that are important. It sounds very simple but actually this is a big change in the way hair has been done in the past. We also charge the client for time rather than the service when it comes to colour. So, if you want both a cut and colour we'll book you in for say an hour or an hour and a half (or maybe three to four hours if you're having a massive colour change and need a longer consultation) and charge you for that time. This allows us to decide how to use that time best rather than booking out separate services with separate people in the salon. It becomes a far more collaborative process when you work like this.

I consider hair colour to fall into one of two camps: obvious statements and 'believable'. A colour statement is something probably quite bold: maybe you want to go a brilliant icy white blonde or perhaps a sugary pastel pink. The second camp, 'believable', is by far the more popular of the two.

A great colour is one that looks as though it really belongs to you and that a colourist hasn't had a hand in creating it. A convincing natural-looking colour is one that complements your skin tone, enhances the colour of your eyes and makes your features come alive. Rarely is that effect achieved with an all-over colour, which is where at-home colour from a box falls short. If you were to look at truly natural, un-dyed hair under a microscope you would see dozens upon dozens of colours; they only read as one colour in real life because our eyes can't distinguish the individual shades without some help. A boxed colour will dye every single one of your hairs the same colour. Yes, it covers greys but the end result is a very flat colour that can't pass as natural. The only time a box dye really gets the job done is if you want to take your hair to a solid jet black.

I do believe that everything is a whole lot simpler if you decide from the get-go whether you are a blonde or have dark hair. Then stick with it. It is never a good idea to change between the two – it causes a lot of damage and the results are never great. I think perhaps because the women we see on our TVs and on social media appear to go from black, to blonde, to violet, to red and back again on the turn of a dime, it leads others to think that these kinds of dramatic colour changes are achievable. What they don't know is that these celebrities are wearing very expensive, very convincing wigs and the only part of it that is 'real' will be along the hairline and the parting.

The role of a colourist is to bring out the best possible version of you and the way they do that is by painting colour onto the hair. A bad colourist is one that sits behind you in the salon and dyes or highlights your hair the same colour from root to tip, rinses you off and sends you on your way. A *great* colourist is one with exceptional technical ability but who also draws outside the lines. Someone who gives you a proper consultation, offers you an opinion and talks you through the possibilities for your hair. When they're actually doing your hair, they're not just absorbed in their work or going through some kind of process, but they are constantly looking in the mirror at you and tailoring your colour by working out where you need more lightness and where you need more darkness.

A brilliant colour is entirely bespoke. Terms like balayage and smudging are bandied about but essentially what you need to know is that your colourist is not adopting a one-size-fits-all approach for your hair. Their Instagram account should serve as their portfolio; if you get a good feeling from their feed, then book yourself in for a consultation. A good colourist can make your hair appear thicker by painting on tones close to your natural shade in

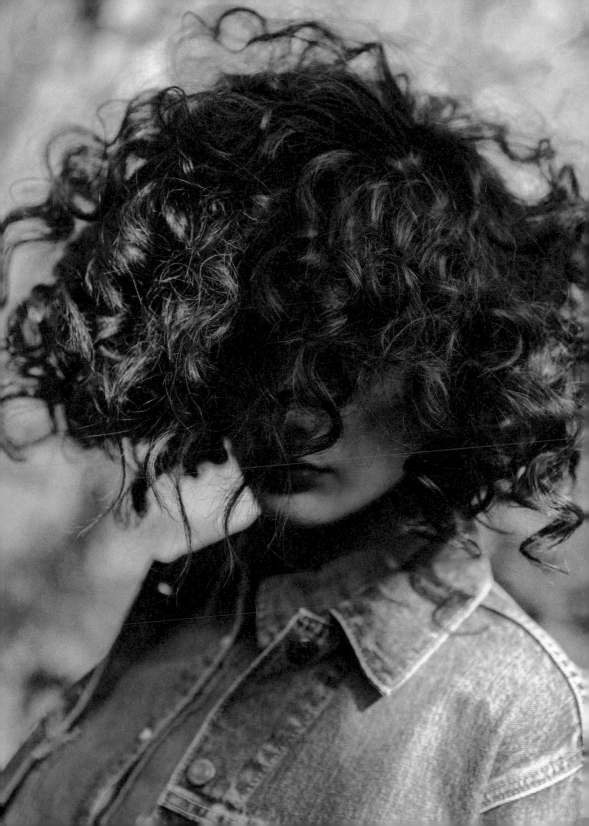

specific places, using a technique that's a bit like *trompe l'œil*; adding some lightness here and some darkness there creates an illusion of bigger hair. The moment you add some variation in colour it adds depth and makes your hair more substantial. Making roots a bit darker and the ends a bit lighter makes the colour look more natural and the regrowth less obvious which actually means that you have to get your colour done less often, saving you some money on appointments in the process. A great colourist – and indeed a great cutter – is akin to an artist in this respect; they are not just going through the motions, they are really looking at you and thinking about placement as they're going.

Unfortunately, there are far too many colourists operating in salons everywhere who don't investigate what a client wants to achieve with their colour; they dye hair in a textbook fashion that's outdated and quite simply doesn't look good. It actually makes me feel quite angry that salons aren't moving things on in terms of colour and demanding more from their colourists.

I don't want you to fall into this trap. Here's how you can avoid it:

Finding a colourist: The best way to find a great colourist is via a recommendation from someone whose colour you love. But don't go on recommendation alone. Check out their Instagram feed to see their handiwork and also who they are inspired by. Next get onto the salon's website and see if their cutters and colourists have their work on there. If they do not have Instagram or their work displayed online then it's a real gamble as to whether you should let them loose on your hair.

Bring pictures: Pictures are not only useful for showing your hairdresser a cut that you like, they also convey what you want from your hair colour.

Communicate: If your colourist doesn't sit down and talk to you about your hair they're probably not someone you should entrust it to. They should ask you questions about what you want to achieve with your colour, whether you want your hair to look thicker, shinier or richer. This is a two-way process. You must be explicit about what you want, what you like and what you really dislike.

Pay attention: I know it's tempting to get lost in a good book or answer all of those pressing emails in your inbox but do try and observe your colourist as well. Are they constantly looking in the mirror at you or are they barely looking in your direction and just routinely applying your colour? If it's the former, you're onto a winner.

DAMAGE CONTROL

Dyeing your hair inevitably results in some damage (though definitely less than in the past) as it has to lift the cuticle layer to allow the colour to penetrate the hair shaft. Lifting your hair to a lighter shade is more damaging than taking it darker. Thankfully there have been some exceptional innovations of late that drastically reduce the damage. Olaplex and L'Oréal Professional Smartbond are in-salon treatments that you can have done during your colour appointment. They work slightly differently but ultimately they protect the hair bonds during the colouring process. They are absolutely brilliant and very well worth using. Not all salons use treatments like this yet, so it is a good idea to check with them when you book your appointment. There is likely to be a further cost for it but in my opinion it is definitely worth it.

AFTERCARE

It's false economy to spend a lot of money in the salon on your hair only to use the wrong products when you get home. Use a shampoo and conditioner that have been specifically formulated to prolong the life-span of colour. Sulphates create a satisfying lather from your shampoo but they also accelerate colour fade. Most colour-safe products are formulated without sulphates so as not to disturb the pigment – they might not lather up as much but they are just as effective. Color Wow Color Security Shampoo is brilliant as it also contains amino acids and proteins that strengthen the hair and help prevent breakage.

Some fading is inevitable after a time, at which point swap to John Frieda Brilliant Brunette or Radiant Red (depending on your colour) which will restore some of its vibrancy until you can next get into the salon. If, however, you're blonde you may notice your colour become brassy after a while. If this is the case use a purple-based shampoo and conditioner to correct the change in tone. John Frieda Sheer Blonde Colour Renew Tone-Correcting Shampoo, TIGI Catwalk Fashionista Violet Shampoo, Bleach Silver Shampoo and Sachajuan Silver Shampoo (despite the names they're purple) are brilliant options.

Lastly, if you have troublesome greys that crop up in between salon appointments buy Color Wow Root Cover Up. It comes in eight shades and looks a little like an eyeshadow palette but if you pat the powder onto your roots and greys with the little brush it will convincingly disguise them. It's really rather brilliant.

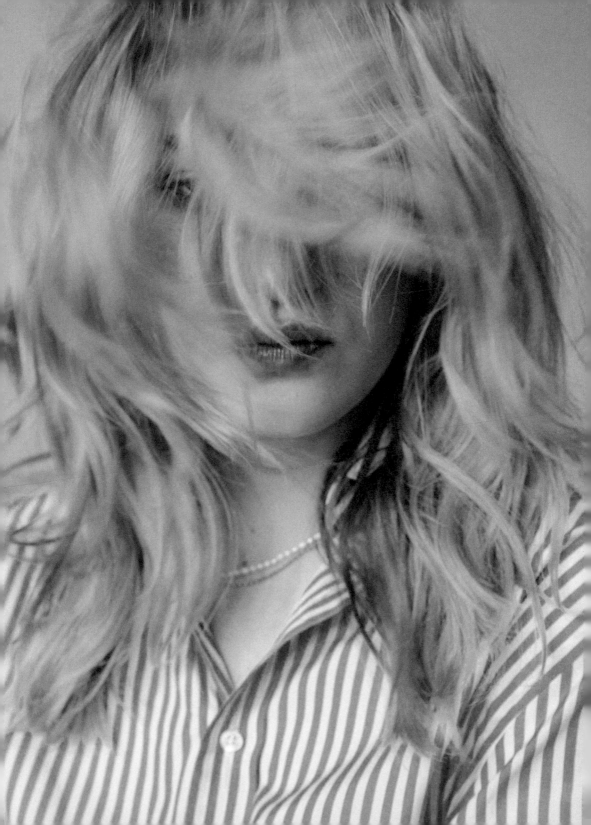

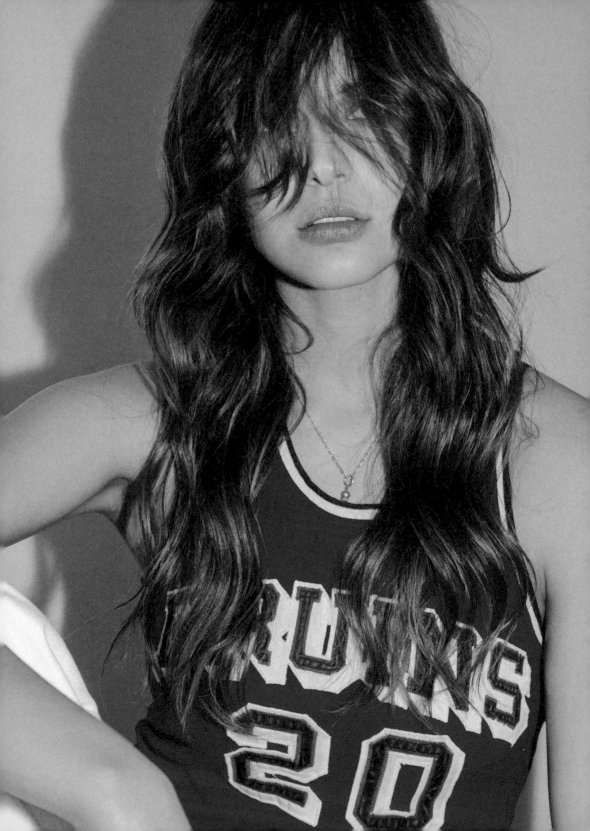

HAIR
ICONS

'The fringe,
the perfect shade,
everything'

Everyone needs to get their inspiration from somewhere. You never want to directly copy someone: for starters it's not original, but also when it comes to your hair a carbon-copy of another person's style may not flatter you in the same way it does them. However, we encourage women to come into Hershesons with inspiration images so that we can see what their likes and dislikes are; a picture is really a brilliant form of communication. And we can't help but notice a few regulars in these inspo pics. The following names crop up time and time again when the women who visit us talk about hair that they love. And we can totally see why . . .

VICTORIA BECKHAM

No one embraces change like Victoria. She has lived much of her adult life in the public eye and so we've all had a front-row seat to her various hair transformations. She really knows how to utilise her hair in a way to define her character; just think back to the bob she debuted in 2006 (which quickly became known as the Pob), the blonde crop she had in 2007 or that incredibly beautiful glossy pixie crop in 2008. Victoria's cut always feel perfect for the moment in time. She's brave in that way. Her hair now is extremely covetable; it's rich and glossy and luxe looking but she is still not afraid to cut some off every now and then. I was working with her on a cover not too long ago and we made an almost spur-of-the-moment decision to cut it shorter. I cut it with a razor so that it just grazed her shoulders and it looked awesome. I can't wait to see where we take her hair next.

SIENNA MILLER

Whether her hair is long and bohemian or cut into a Bad Bob, Sienna's hair is the ultimate in hair goals. When people come into the salon and ask for a fringe, nine times out of ten they have a picture of Sienna with them. I kind of think of her as a modern Brigitte Bardot; there's something nicely rock 'n' roll and carefree about her – her look is very nonchalant.

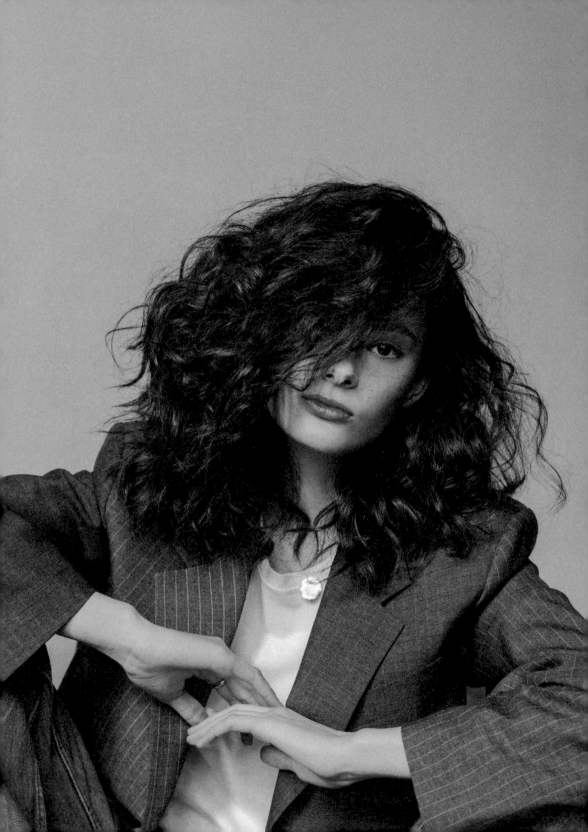

RIHANNA

Rihanna is some kind of chameleon; her look evolves almost on a weekly basis. I suppose she is kind of like Madonna in the way she skilfully plays with and updates her appearance. Some of her most famous hairstyles – such as the brilliant blonde Farrah Fawcett-inspired number a few years back and the Little Mermaid flaming locks she had for the 2011 Met Gala in New York – are either wigs or extensions. Rihanna knows how to have fun with her hair and embraces traditional Afro hairstyles and characteristics like Bantu Knots and baby hairs but at the same time loves an undercut and retro Victory Rolls. It's never a dull moment with Rihanna.

GISELE BÜNDCHEN

My first big break was working with Gisele in Sardinia on a campaign for Missoni. The look was classic Gisele: bronzed sandy skin, pared-back make-up and masses upon masses of sun-kissed beachy waves. Those waves have come to define Gisele's style and often when women come into the salon with reference images for their highlights or cut, they'll be of Gisele. Her appeal is huge and despite having officially retired from modelling she is still a globally recognised modern beauty icon – and for good reason.

ZOE KRAVITZ

How is it possible for one person to be so cool? But then again, is it any wonder when your mother is the actress Lisa Bonet? Zoe once told an interviewer that she has always found her hair's kinky texture to be a challenge, but you wouldn't know it from the number of outstanding styles she has rocked over the last few years. Zoe is vocal about her love for braids – whether they're fine or boxy – and doesn't shy away from colour. On one occasion she paired her bleached hair with a radical buzz cut – the result was so delicate and pixie-like. Seriously cool.

KATE MOSS

Kate Moss is all things – hair inspiration, fashion inspiration and make-up inspiration – for so many women. Looking back through her library – so to speak – is like taking a lesson in hair evolution. At one time she was the definition of grunge, then she became this modern Brigitte Bardot, then she moved on to this amazing short elfin haircut and then there was that blonde wedge cut of the early noughties. I think some of her best looks were in pictures taken by Patrick Demarchelier quite early on in her career. Now she has this very British sensibility about her that says she doesn't want to look as though she has tried too hard. Kate can do no wrong.

DIANA ROSS

I don't think anyone has ever, or will ever, work an Afro like Diana Ross. Her hair is the stuff of legends and quite rightly so. For Diana it has always been a case of the bigger the better as far as her hair is concerned, even back when she was wearing it in a bob. In 1969 Diana gave us one of the most memorable hair moments of all time when she performed on Broadway with the Supremes and the Temptations with a flower-adorned wig to rival Marie Antoinette. It was out of the world.

BRIGITTE BARDOT

Brigitte Bardot's hairstyles in the sixties are as desirable now as they were then. Whether it was her sex-kitten peek-a-boo fringe, or undone up-do, cutesy pigtails or playful ponytail, they are truly timeless looks. Back then she was also the unofficial queen of the hair accessory and loved to wear wide headbands and oversized bows, which, funnily enough, we have seen a lot of over the last couple of seasons at the shows. And if you're looking for the ultimate soft and creamy shade of blonde, hers was it.

GOLDIE HAWN

In *Shampoo*, *Overboard* and *Bird on a Wire* Goldie Hawn dished up some of the best movies of the seventies, eighties and nineties and her hair was bloody brilliant in each and every one of them. Her look in *Shampoo* has to be my favourite: the fringe, the perfect shade of blonde, everything. She has never deviated too far from her signature choppy blonde hair. She knows what works and she sticks with it. Never change, Goldie!

JANE BIRKIN

When it comes to Jane it's about that fringe. Despite being born in England, Jane is famed for her Parisian sense of style, a style that she passed on to her daughters Kate Barry, Charlotte Gainsbourg and Lou Doillon. The look she is best known for is her mid-length brunette hair and full fringe – it's such a French look, very simple and naive. It's a very sweet style and one that women of all ages still come back to time and time again.

GRACE JONES

Sure, she was a Bond Girl but Grace Jones was a Bond Girl with a difference; she was fierce and more than a match for 007. At the time it was incredibly rare to see a woman be so bold and so different in the way she looked. I post a lot of inspirational images to my Instagram account of actresses, singers and models who have hair that I think is utterly incredible. Looking back through my feed I've noticed that I tend to post images of women who are strong and a little androgynous. This is exactly how I see Grace. Her graphic, not-to-be-messed-with, razor-sharp box cut was daring then and it still is – plus, she is not only a hair inspiration but also a millinery muse as over the years she has worn the most outlandish and theatrical headwear designed by Philip Treacy. She is iconic.

GEORGIA MAY JAGGER

Granted, with parents like Mick Jagger and Jerry Hall, Georgia May Jagger was always going to be a trend-setter. She has a very unique ability to carry off a thoroughly vintage, old-Hollywood aesthetic with its cascading waves and bold red lips. But she's also somewhat of a chameleon and can swap retro glam for boho seventies with the snip of a fringe. Georgia May's seventies parted Curtain Fringe is up there with the best.

THE CURL GIRLS

The best curls to have ever existed belonged to Kim Basinger, Nicole Kidman and Julia Roberts in the eighties. Fact. While each offered a different take on curls – Kim's were undeniably sexy, Nicole's youthful and naive, and Julia was very much the girl next door – their styles have managed to stand the test of time. Perms are becoming increasingly popular again at Hershesons and we have spent some time in refining our methods so that the end result is cool and modern and about as far from poodle as you can get. I think we're going to be seeing lots more of these types of curls.

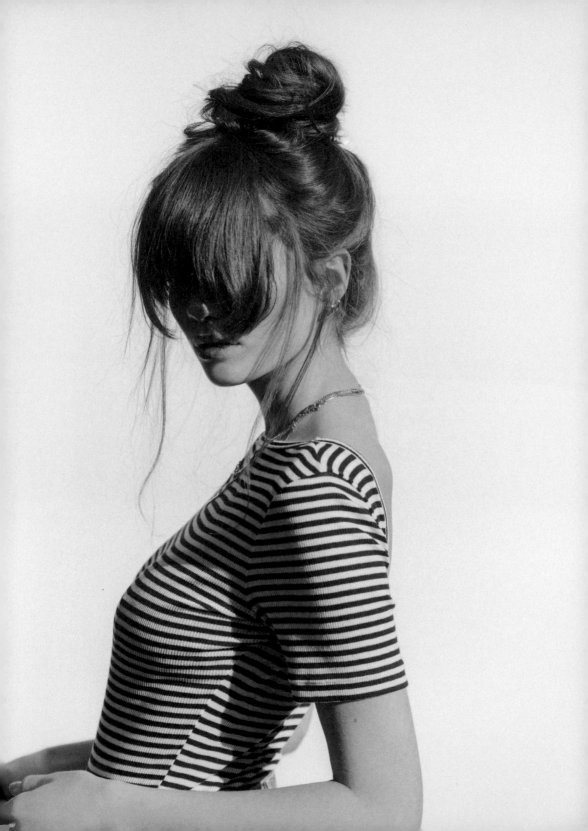

COOL
SPECIAL
OCCASION
HAIR

'Fantastically memorable, show-stopping gorgeous hair without clichés'

There are occasions when we are expected to scrub up, when we need – and want – to look like the best possible version of ourselves. But special occasion hair can be in itself a trap – a trap for good taste, that is. There is evidently still an outdated prescribed school of hairdressing in force where 'special occasion' translates as crispy ringlets, uncomfortable chignons, stiff-as-a-board backcombing and more diamante hair accessories than you can throw a stick at.

I think special occasion hair means a very different thing today – or at least it *should* do. Whether you're going to a formal dinner, a party or even your own wedding it is, as ever, important to look like yourself and not like a caricature. You can have fantastically memorable, show-stopping gorgeous hair without falling foul of fancy hair clichés, and it is more than possible to look classic without looking too 'done'. The other upside of a more relaxed approach to special occasion hair (aside from a thoroughly modern and beautiful style that will make you smile when you look back through photographs) is that they tend to wear well all the way through the main event to the after-party and, ahem, the morning after.

So, forget everything you thought you knew about appropriate event-worthy hair and adopt one, or all, of the following.

THE CLASSIC WAVE

A glossy wave that falls over one eye is unbelievably glamorous, which is why it is the look *du jour* of every awards season and, as a result, has seen many a red carpet (think Veronica Lake). This style of retro wave is just made for a wedding – even your own – or a formal black-tie event. Despite being a definite look, modern glossy waves should still look luscious and touchable and a far cry from their stiff forties predecessors.

You need: Styling cream, hairdryer with nozzle, comb, medium-sized round-barrelled ceramic brush, medium-sized curling tong, mixed-bristle brush, hairspray and hairgrips (optional).

Step 1: Apply a styling cream containing heat protection to damp, freshly washed hair.

Step 2: Rough-dry your hair using just your hands until it is 95 per cent dry. Do not use a brush at this point; you will just be wasting your time and causing unnecessary stress to your hair.

Step 3: Use your comb to create that all-important side parting. It doesn't hugely matter where you place your parting so long as it's off-centre.

Step 4: Now you must blow-dry your hair. Section your hair into chunks around three inches wide and wrap them around your brush (which should be placed underneath the section of hair). Aim the airflow from your hairdryer directly at the brush as you pull it down through your hair. Work your way steadily around your entire head. You don't need to worry about aiming the air at your roots, or trying to create volume, as these waves look better when the top section of the hair is flatter.

Step 5: The only place you *do* want some volume is the very front section that sweeps across your eye. A little lift here looks really sexy. When you're blow-drying the front section, aim your hairdryer directly at your roots from underneath the brush – this will create a little height.

Step 6: Time to tong. Use a medium-barrelled curling tong and work in sections a couple of inches wide. Make sure you place the tong underneath the section of hair and wrap around it from above, leaving the roots out so they remain flat.

Step 7: Hold the hair around the tong for about twenty seconds before removing it and capturing the curl in the palm of your hand. If time is of the essence just allow a few seconds for the curl to cool before releasing it. If, however, you have a bit more time on your hands you can create a more pronounced wave by capturing the curl as you release the tong and securing it in its coiled shape against your head with a sectioning clip. Once you have done all of your hair like this, you can leave the clips in while you finish getting dressed and do your make-up.

Step 8: Once your hair is down again it will look very curly indeed but don't worry, we're about to soften everything. Brush through the hair with a flat brush to soften the curls and bring the waves together.

Step 9: Rub a little more styling cream between your hands and smooth over the waves to take down any fluff, add shine and encourage them to come together as a kind of waterfall. The top sections of your hair around your parting need to stay quite flat, so tuck the side that is not going over your eye behind your ear and give everything a mist of hairspray.

Tip: If the hair behind your ear keeps coming forward you can easily keep it in place with a discreetly placed hairgrip.

THE 'NEW' UP-DO

Up-dos are still a perfect accompaniment to a special occasion but they must not look contrived otherwise you may well look as though you're attending a Sweet Sixteen rather than a grown-up soirée. This is an up-do I recently created for Victoria Beckham for – funnily enough – a special occasion, so I know it works. It's up but it's a little undone and quite relaxed – in fact, it's about as far from contrived as you can get – so it's the perfect counterpoint to an elegant dress.

You need: Styling cream, medium-sized curling tong, mixed-bristle brush, hair elastic, hairgrips and hairspray.

Step 1: This up-do all comes down to the texture – there must be plenty of movement in your hair. Work a little styling cream with heat protection through dry hair to prep it for the oncoming heat.

Step 2: Tong your hair in no particular fashion. The hair is, after all, going up but this step is crucial. Work your way around your head, tonging random sections of no specific width.

Step 3: I truly believe that your hands are your best styling tool and it's time to put them to use. Get your hands in your hair and shake everything up.

Step 4: To create some height around your crown use a mixed-bristle brush to back-brush a few sections of hair. To do this all you need to do is put the brush against the underneath of your hair a few centimetres from your roots and brush the hair backwards towards your head. Only do this in one direction and not frantically back and forth. This is a much gentler alternative to the backcombing that dominated the eighties and it is much easier to brush out at the end of the evening.

Step 5: Pull your hair into a ponytail that's above the occipital bone (the bone at the back of your head just above the top of your neck) and tie it off with a hair elastic.

Step 6: Take hold of the ponytail and fold it into a loop around your fingers. Flatten it against your head, over the base of your ponytail, to create a kind of flattened bun. Now pin it in place with hairgrips.

Step 7: Work some more styling cream between your hands and use your fingers to rough up the hair around your hairline so everything looks very soft. Once you're happy with it, mist with hairspray.

Tip: The more 'worn' this hair looks the better so if you know you won't have time to fix your hair during the evening then this is the style for you.

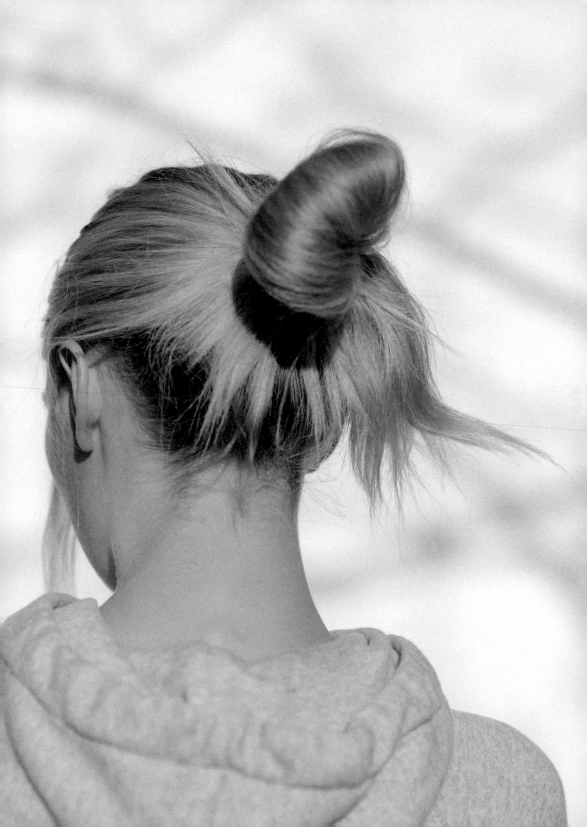

THE PARTY PONY

In a way, the style of ponytail – whether you wear it low or high on your head, whether it's dishevelled or pristine and glossy – is kind of irrelevant. A ponytail, in any guise, can make for spectacular special occasion hair and it's the ultimate customisable hairstyle. Where your ponytail sits says a lot about your character; wear it sleek and low when you're feeling the need for something graphic with an Armani feel, or higher up on your head and loosely contained with pieces falling about your face if you want to look more ethereal and romantic. Ponytails love accessories and a black velvet ribbon tied in a bow around its base looks stunning.

Special occasion hair should not always be about a hair statement; it's sometimes just about bringing balance to a look. You don't want everything to 'shout', and if what you're wearing is elaborate or vintage you do not want to put vintage hair, or a lot of hair, with it. This is why a ponytail is so great because it brings balance to strong fashion statements.

You need: Styling cream, mixed-bristle brush, hairband or hair elastic and hairspray.

Step 1: Smooth some styling cream through dry hair to reduce frizz.

Step 2: Use a mixed-bristle brush to brush your hair back into a ponytail. Gather the hair wherever you want the base of your ponytail to be and tie it off with either a thin hairband or a piece of elastic. Bungee-style elastics (hair elastics with hooks at either end, which are often easier to use) are great if you want something really neat and tight, and they're also good if you want to guarantee your hair stays put all night – if I'm getting someone ready for the red carpet I will always use a bungee elastic.

Step 3: If you are creating something sleek use your mixed-bristle brush to smooth the surface of the hair. However, if you are after something looser use your thumb and forefinger to pinch and soften the hair in places and pull a few strands loose from the ponytail.

Step 4: Regardless of whether your ponytail is smooth and sleek or thoughtfully destroyed, mist everything with hairspray to set.

Tip: You can really sharpen your features – a mini facelift of sorts – just by pulling a small section of hair either side of your head by your temple tightly backwards and securing into your ponytail.

THE SWANK

The Swank is an up-do we have on the menu at Hershesons. It's inspired by Hilary Swank's sleek bun that she wore to the 2005 Oscars when she picked up the Best Actress award for *Million Dollar Baby*. It's super chic, lady-like, unbelievably glamorous, but still soft and shiny and elegant. From the front, the Swank looks very ordinary, very proper, but the moment you turn your head and reveal the back you're unleashing the detail. This is what makes this style so modern. To me, the Swank is about as complicated an up-do should get – and that's not very much at all.

You need: Styling cream, comb, hairgrips, hairspray and vintage hair comb (optional).

Step 1: Prepare dry hair with some styling cream to reduce any frizz and give some staying power to the style.

Step 2: Use a comb to create a side parting on whichever side suits you best. It doesn't have to be a particularly low parting, just off the centre of your head will do.

Step 3: Using an imaginary line from your crown, down the back of your head to the nape of your neck, split your hair into two sections. Now take those two sections and tie them together loosely as if you were tying a shoelace; so cross one over the other, and then take the underneath piece up and over and into the gap between the two. Depending on the length

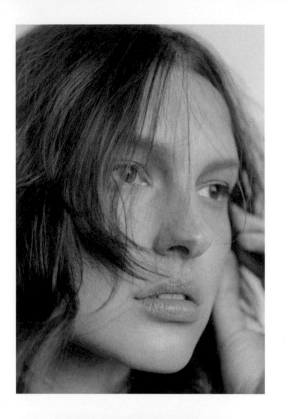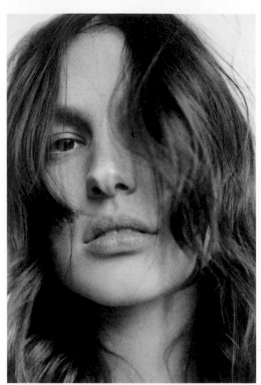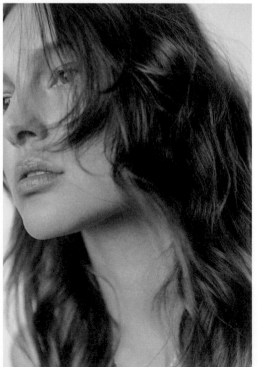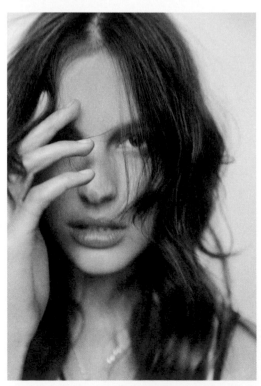

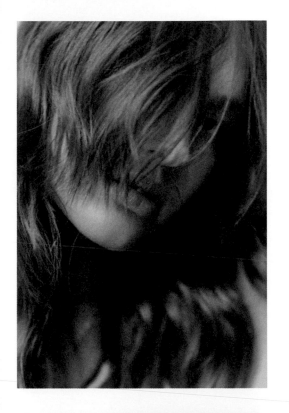
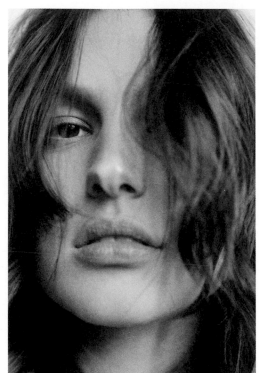
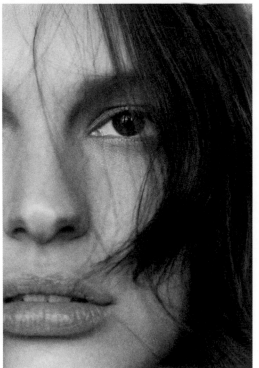
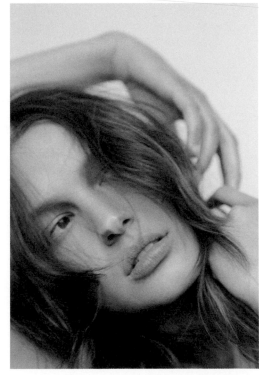

of your hair, repeat again so you end up with a double knot. You're quickly building something that, on the surface, looks quite intricate. Don't panic, this will come out really easily at the end of the night.

Step 4: If you have a little tail of hair poking out from the knot, twist it to reduce it in size and then tuck it up underneath the knot and secure in place with some grips. Add some more grips around the rest of the knot until it feels very secure.

Step 5: Now it needs to be destroyed a little so use your fingers to loosen the knot in places so the whole thing feels a little bit more effortless. It doesn't need to be perfect, that's the whole point of this look.

Step 6: Set everything with a mist of hairspray.

Tip: The Swank makes for a beautiful bridal 'do' and can be dressed up even further with a vintage hair comb tucked into the top of the knot.

A LESSON IN BRIDAL HAIR

Perhaps the grandest special occasion of your lifetime is your own wedding. Here's how to get your hair right:

Now is not the time to experiment with a radical new look (remember, those photographs will last a lifetime). On your wedding day the aim is to look like a more polished version of you; the person that your partner fell in love with.

Bring balance to your overall look. Just like any other kind of special occasion hair, this is the role of your hairstyle on your wedding day. If you have a very intricate dress or a huge train, your hair shouldn't set out as competition – instead it should soften the effect. Similarly, if your dress is simplicity at its best, you can afford to make more of a statement with your hair.

Don't wear ALL the hair accessories. Less is more. You don't have to wear the barrette, *and* the tiara, *and* the flowers, *and* the veil. It's just far, far too much. Pick one.

Think of it as your own red carpet. What are you going to love to see in the photographs afterwards?

Be realistic about the cost of getting your hair done. I know it seems that as soon as you mention the word 'wedding' the prices of things rocket but in the case of your hair there are very good reasons why it costs more. If you want your long-term hairdresser to leave the salon, travel to your venue and do your hair, your mum's hair and your entire bridal party then, yes, unfortunately that is likely to cost a fair bit of money. The stylist has to factor time in away from the salon, the travel expenses, the travel time, the time to prepare their kit and the time spent on trial sessions. The cost is likely to be somewhere around double what you would spend to see them in the salon.

Think about what the weather is likely to be. A few years ago I styled Keira Knightley's hair for the UK premiere of her movie *The Imitation Game*. Her Valentino dress was very intricate so I kept her hair very simple in comparison with just a few glossy waves, and I went easy on the product because I wanted her hair to move and come to life as she walked the red carpet. By the time she got to the event the heavens had opened and the wind picked up. Wind can destroy a hairstyle but because everything was very relaxed and soft the wind just picked up a few strands and blew them across her face. The effect was actually rather beautiful and not surprisingly it was those shots that got picked up in the papers the following morning.

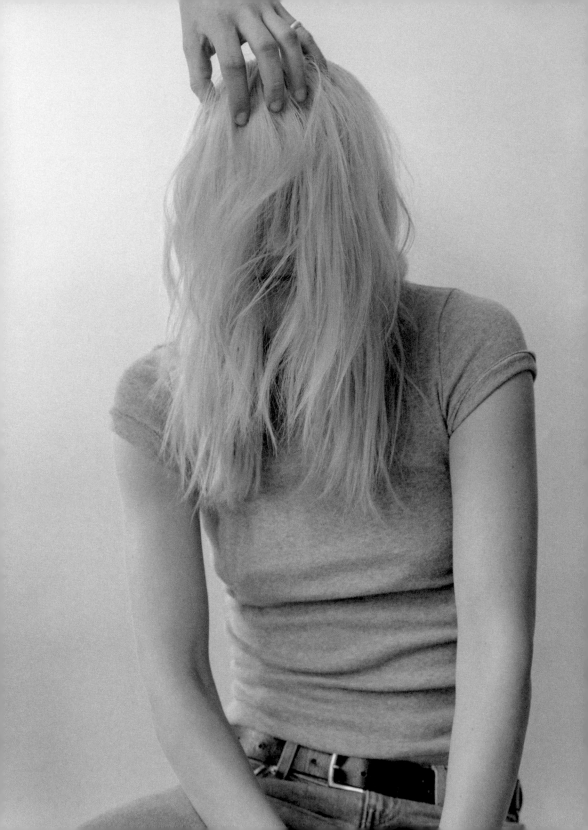

THE
SECRETS
OF
SESSION
HAIR

'Elnett and
your fingers can
work magic in
an instant'

I got into session styling (essentially styling hair on-set or on location) almost as soon as I started in the industry, probably before I was even technically qualified if I'm honest. When I was about sixteen or seventeen I was asked by our PR company to go to Kentish Town in North London and do the hair for a test shoot. Up until then I had assisted my dad on things but this shoot was really the first time I took the reins and styled hair for a picture myself. That shoot was the start of everything.

Being a session hairdresser is a completely different job from being a salon hairdresser. The only thing they have in common, of course, is that you're playing with hair but that's where the similarities end. The salon experience is about transformation, it's about building relationships with your clients and it's about communication. Being on-set is really about making something that's essentially three-dimensional become alive in a two-dimensional way. Let me tell you, that's a very different skill set.

A photographer once said to me, 'As a hairdresser, you're working with something real and moving and you have to be able to see how it is going to sit as a graphic on a page.' And that is essentially what session hairdressing is. It's all about creating a picture, and hair, much more so than make-up – and probably as much as the fashion –really dictates what that picture will look like. The job of a hairdresser on-set is to communicate who this 'woman' is, who she hangs out with, where she is from and what she likes to do – it's building a personality. As much as we create hair it's very much about creating characters – in fact, it is as much about characters as it is about hair.

It's the little nuances that say so much in an image. Where you position a ponytail, where you carve out a parting – they're their own cultural 'clues' that suggest the feel of the story is, for example, very American or very European. If you can imagine that something so small can say so much, then you can begin to imagine what bigger style choices, like curls or hair colour, are saying. The person flicking through the magazine and stopping to look at the picture may not realise it but they are 'reading' that image, picking up on subtle clues in order to understand it.

It's kind of a given that when the hair is not right, nothing is right. If a shoot is not heading in the right direction, the hair is always the first thing to change because most of the time the clothes we're shooting are already locked in beforehand and so they cannot change. If you want to add coolness, sexiness, toughness or boyishness, the most reliable way to do so is to change up the hair. Naturally, this means that the hairdresser is usually the one who has to take it on the chin and get to work.

I was taught very early on in my career that hair doesn't really happen in the wardrobe – or the area in the studio dedicated to dressing, hair and make-up – the idea that you come into the set, do the hair and make-up in the morning and then the model goes off to be shot doesn't work in reality. Most of my work actually comes to life on-set in front of the camera. I always have a little table standing by the set with whatever I might need and in between shots I will adjust the model's hair; whether that's a little bit of backcombing, or adding some shape or a hairpiece, it really doesn't matter.

Another huge difference between what I do on-set and what I do in the salon is that on-set I'm creating something that's only going to last for a moment; the model doesn't have to live with it once she has stepped outside the studio. Because of that there is a lot of trickery involved to get that 'moment' just so.

There's always a wind machine on-set but I also carry a couple of things in my kit to help us nail the look. A hairdresser's on-set staple is a board that we use to create just a gentle waft of air rather than a full-on wind. A waft is enough to just lift the hair and make it appear thicker and fuller – even without adding a hairpiece. Giving this kind of movement to the hair really makes that 3D-to-2D transition a lot easier and that final image look vibrant and alive even though it's a still. Most stylists now also carry an actual leaf blower in their kit – the kind you use in the garden and buy in a hardware store – 'wind' is a very big deal in this business (you think I'm kidding). I often have very in-depth conversations with fellow stylist Syd Hayes about wind and waft with regards to hair. Mine is by a brand called

Makita and it's a full-on piece of gardening equipment. Needless to say, it usually attracts some attention when I check my bags in at the airport on my way to a shoot.

Every shoot is unique to some extent (which is why it pays to always be prepared). If we're not shooting a hair story – and it's either a single model or maybe a personality like an actress – then the look comes together after a discussion with the photographer, the stylist and the make-up artist. On shoots like this, I'm just the hairdresser and part of a team. Not every shoot is about a major hair moment that's going to dominate an entire page, and when it's not you have to know when to pull everything back and leave the hair a little more subtle or pared down than you normally would. After all, the hair has to be in harmony with everything else that is going to appear in that image. It's at times such as these that, as the hairdresser, you actually do very little and, bizarrely, it requires a lot of confidence to do little on-set and not feel as though you *have* to make a statement with the hair. If, however, we're shooting a hair story for a magazine – where the hair is different in every picture – there is more pressure on me to come up with the concept and choose the team.

How the picture evolves really depends on who the photographer is, what you're doing, whether you're in the studio or on location, whether you have just the one model or lots of them. Some photographers love lots of movement and want to shoot the hair at every angle. Others, more traditional studio photographers, are looking for that one angle so it really doesn't matter how the hair that's not in the frame looks. Either way, most of the magic happens on-set, in front of the camera, and it can all come together very quickly.

Location shoots can be pretty interesting. My first big break was a Missoni campaign job with Gisele Bündchen. We were shooting in Sardinia on these huge boulders that looked like Death Valley and we had to trek what felt like miles to get to them.

Since then I have had to work in some weird and wonderful places. I remember trying to cut hair with very little light at 4 a.m. in a petrol service station in Dubai. I have had to do battle with the winds on the Yorkshire Moors and style Courtney Love's hair while we were both in a swimming pool in Ibiza. There have been jobs in Morocco, the Canary Islands, LA and Albuquerque, on salt flats in California, a glacier in Norway, a haunted house on the outskirts of Paris and a cemetery in New York. For the twenty-fifth anniversary of *Dazed* magazine we shot Gigi Hadid in the *Dazed* offices where she was basically smashing the place up and chucking laptops on the floor. And then there was that time I worked on a Kylie Minogue music video and had to get 150 extras – plus Kylie of course – ready for camera.

I have certainly racked up some air miles over the years but it has not always been plain sailing. One time, after flying to New York for a job, my kit didn't arrive. I landed at 10 p.m. and was due on set first thing in the morning. I had to pinch the hairdryer from the hotel, borrow some brushes from a friend and turn up on-set with very little else. The irony is, I'm a very particular person and like to travel with absolutely everything in my kit just in case it should be needed. I travel with a collection of about two hundred wigs, fifty different shades of hair extensions, Geisha hair padding and a wig-making kit and telescopic stand so I can work on wigs wherever I am in the world. It was way out of my comfort zone to turn up to a job with so little.

This kind of profession requires some out-of-this-world organisational skills and you need a team around you who understand the way you work. My assistants tend to stay with me for between two and four years and I always have at least one with me on a job – sometimes more if the job demands it. A lot of the guys in the salon have assisted me at one time or another and I really feel that session work is an invaluable training ground for new or very young hairdressers. Working on fashion shoots helps you develop a good level of taste and to understand what's vulgar, what's ironic, what's in good taste and what looks cheap. Every one of these things has a time and a place and the experience you gain on-set teaches you when each should come into play; it teaches you to form an opinion.

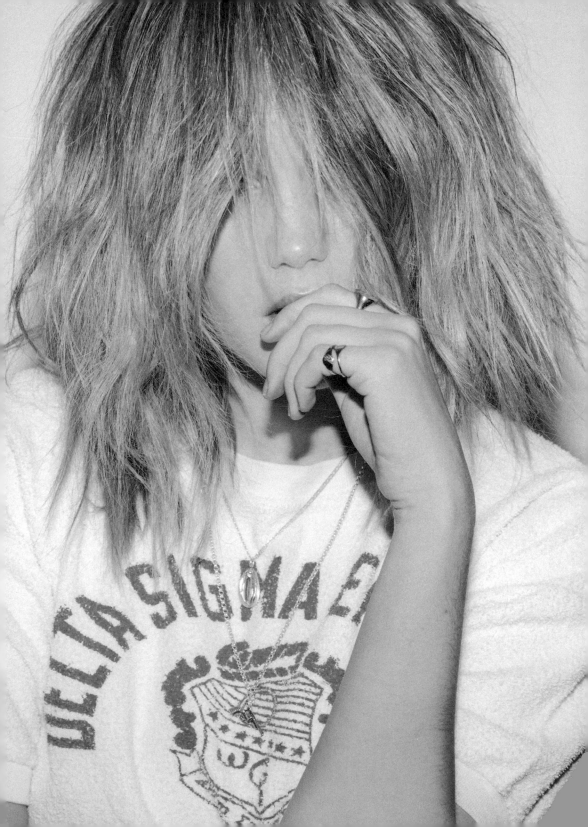

One of the things I remember Guido Palau telling me when I was starting out was, 'You have got to walk onto the set with an opinion and ideas. Whether those ideas are right or wrong, is not as important as showing that you are bringing something to the table.' It was invaluable advice.

Those first few years on-set you're really just trying to get to grips with the basics; how light affects the hair, when to speak up and when to just kind of nod your head and say yes. Knowing how to navigate being on-set is not something you learn overnight. I spent the first five years or so of my session career working at an incredibly high level when, in all honesty, I don't think I was particularly ready for it. In those early days I worked a lot with David Sims who is an enormously successful fashion photographer. I think of the couple of years I spent with him as an apprenticeship of sorts because he knows hair so well and he knows what works on a page. Everything I learned from him made me a much better hairdresser. It has taken me the best part of twenty years to get to a point where photographers look to me not just for my hair skills but for my opinion. Now, after a shoot, I feel as though my opinion was wanted and needed, and that I have really contributed to a story. That's a great feeling and a really nice position to be in.

HOW TO LOOK GREAT
IN A PICTURE

Elnett and your fingers can work magic in an instant. Mist your hair from a distance to bring some life and texture to it and then really get your hands in there to build a little body at the roots or add shape to your hair.

Natural moments always look better than posed-for photographs. Make sure you get a few shots (whether you're taking a selfie or getting someone to take your picture). Move around a little, change the direction of your glance or the shape of your smile. The camera is far more likely to capture the perfect moment like this.

Angle is important. Shooting from a slightly elevated angle is always more flattering whereas shooting from below makes you look a little bigger in the frame.

A ring flash always helps. There are plenty of clip-on ring lights or selfie lights that you can add to your camera phone that will cast a soft-focus and more flattering light on you.

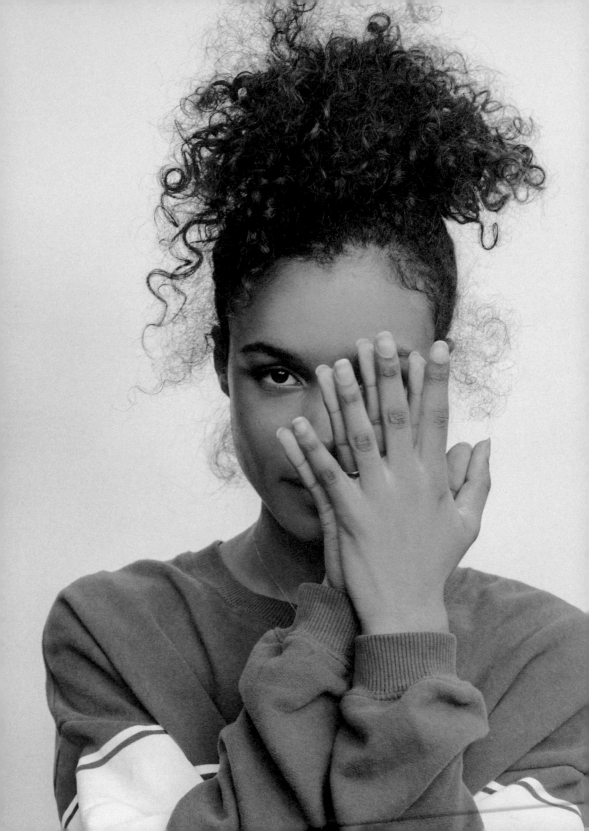

SHOW TIME: WHAT REALLY GOES ON BACKSTAGE

'When everything comes together it is just magic'

I can't help but liken a Fashion Week backstage area with a professional kitchen. Sound mad? Bear with me. In most professional kitchens (and I'm of course basing my experience entirely on Gordon Ramsay's *Hell's Kitchen* television programme here) the head chef designs the menu and then oversees his team of chefs as they execute his vision. Then, once everything has been plated up, the head chef inspects the dishes and makes any final tweaks on the pass. Designing the hair and producing a look for a show is exactly the same process.

I learned this way of managing a show from backstage legend Guido Palau back in the day when I was assisting. Assisting Guido was such an exciting time; I worked on shows for Valentino, Chloé, Sonia Rykiel and Alexander McQueen. It was very rare that he actually did much with the hair at all when we were at the show; his hard work came in days – possibly a week – before when he designed the hair in the test appointment with the designer. If you get sucked into working on one model at a show you can easily lose sight of what's happening around you and it's almost impossible to keep on top of things. That's when shit can hit the fan and things go downhill pretty quickly. I do a lot more work at the pass, that final line-up, just before the girl takes to the catwalk – it's then that I can make a few final tweaks like tucking some hair behind an ear, or strategically covering an eye with a wave, or adding some teasing at the crown. This is when you dial the hair up or dial it down, when you push an element a little further and everything comes alive. Of course, in order to work this way you need an incredible team who you trust implicitly to realise your vision. Thankfully, my team are out-of-the-park awesome and 100 per cent an extension of me.

The test is really when a show hairdresser earns their money. Depending on the designer, the test (essentially an opportunity for the stylist, make-up artist and hairdresser to come together to design all the components of the show that will fit around the fashion collection) usually takes place a couple of days or, sometimes, a week before the show date. We'll see some or all of the clothes that are going to be in the show, see the lighting and hear the music for the first time. Lighting – whether the show is lit from above or from the side – is so important and the music is probably even *more* important; the soundtrack really sets the tone of the show. The test is such a vital part of everything – not least because this is when we decide on what we're doing with the hair, but also because this is when I start building a world of make-believe.

The designer is, after all, creating his or her collection with a very specific woman in mind. They know exactly who *their* woman is and how to portray her so it's important that we reflect that aesthetic with the hair and make-up. Typically, I'll arrive to the test – mammoth kit in tow, naturally – and the designer will have pictures and references to show us their thinking and inspirations behind the collection they have created. Some designers are brilliant communicators and some, not so much, so it's really anyone's guess as to whether there will be a single image to show the designer's creative thinking or an entire wall of images and references depicting the intricacies of this character that we have to create and bring to life. The job of the hair and make-up artist is to decipher everything we see at the test and manifest it in a complete look. At times, it's a real challenge.

It's at the test where I will see the model casting for the first time. Over the last few years casting has really become one of the most vital components of any show. The models booked to walk the catwalk have to completely sum up the style and mood of the collection, conveying who the designer is and who they want to be. Look at the Victoria's Secret line-up, for example; the girls they cast in the fashion show are all overtly sexy – even before going through hair and make-up – and that speaks volumes about the clothes they are wearing. On the opposite end of the spectrum you have the Parisian 'design collective' Vetements – who are all about streetwear, hoodies and denim and basically anything else that you wouldn't consider to be stereotypical high-end fashion – where the casting is far edgier, a little cooler and the models all have a touch of something unusual about them. Traditionally, the designer Jean-Paul Gaultier is the king of casting; the girls he books for his shows sum up his vision to a Tee.

It is more and more likely now that a girl will be cast in a show because she has something unique and unquantifiable about her; maybe she has a huge mass of natural curls or maybe she's covered in freckles. Models used to all look the same, but now – refreshingly – they are celebrated for their differences. Just look at Canadian model Winnie Harlow who rose through the ranks of *America's Next Top Model*; she has vitiligo (a disorder that results in patches of white, pigment-free skin) on her face and body which just adds to what makes her beautiful. As hairdressers we are not being asked so much any more to produce an army of identical models where everyone is singing from the same hymn sheet – instead the look is much, much more individual. This turn of events is so interesting to me because really this kind of freedom has never existed in the shows before. I think it's a sign of the times; women are less likely to want to look as though they belong to a particular tribe, and instead everyone wants to have something unique that sets them apart from everyone else.

The job of a hairdresser on a show is to give a sensibility to the character of the woman the show is centred around. I spend a lot of time on the test thinking about who this woman is, what she looks like, her age, where she lives, how she walks, where she's from, who she's inspired by, where she hangs out and what kind of music she's likely to listen to. It's my job to provide some context and help bring the collection to life. You do this on a shoot too but I think this process is even more crucial when creating hair for a show. The clothes tell a story and the hair and make-up message is really there to reinforce that.

Ironically, all of this time spent conjuring up this woman, studying inspiration images and castings, and hours working and tweaking hair in the test can ultimately boil down to something as seemingly simple as a ponytail, but that innocuous ponytail could be a defining piece of the puzzle that brings context to the whole show. Or it is just as likely to culminate in an ornate wig that has to be custom dyed. Nine times out of ten, the look we decide upon at the test will be the look we're going to create backstage on the day. Occasionally there'll be a call afterwards from the designer if they're unsure about an element or want to change something up but that, thankfully, is pretty uncommon.

On the day I'll have a team of between twenty and twenty-five stylists. They have all been working with me for a number of years so we all know how each other ticks and we have our routine nailed down. We'll be set up backstage about three hours before show time – backstage is like a well-oiled machine with each component coming together in synch to get the show off on time. In that window each model has to go through hair, make-up, nails, dressing and a run-through, so there's no time for anything to go wrong and every single person has to pull their weight in order for things to run without a hitch.

Sometimes the hair can be very complicated and time-consuming. I remember doing a show in Milan that required dreadlocks for every model. We spent the entire flight to Italy, until 4 a.m., rubbing hair extensions with our hands to create these dreadlocks. At another show for Jil Sander we had around forty male models, each with longish skater-boy hair, and the brief was to give each one a haircut to turn them into a kind of replica of Steve McQueen. You might think that as men they wouldn't give a shit about their hair but this was the noughties and every male model had grown his hair long. We almost had a riot on our hands.

Depending on the complexity of the hair we're creating I will either demo the look to the team on the morning of the show or we will run through everything the day before so that we can maximise the time we have on the day. If the look is quite complicated and involves various steps I might split my team up so they are each responsible for a different step in the process, a bit like a factory production line. But – as is the way with more and more shows these days – we're often doing a more individual look for each girl and working with her own hair texture and quirks. If that's the case then the model will stay with one stylist throughout the process. You might think that it's easier to just do whatever each girl's hair requires but the truth is, doing something more defined and prescriptive is a whole lot easier because there is a definitive formula to follow with each girl and so there's less room for error or misinterpretation of the brief.

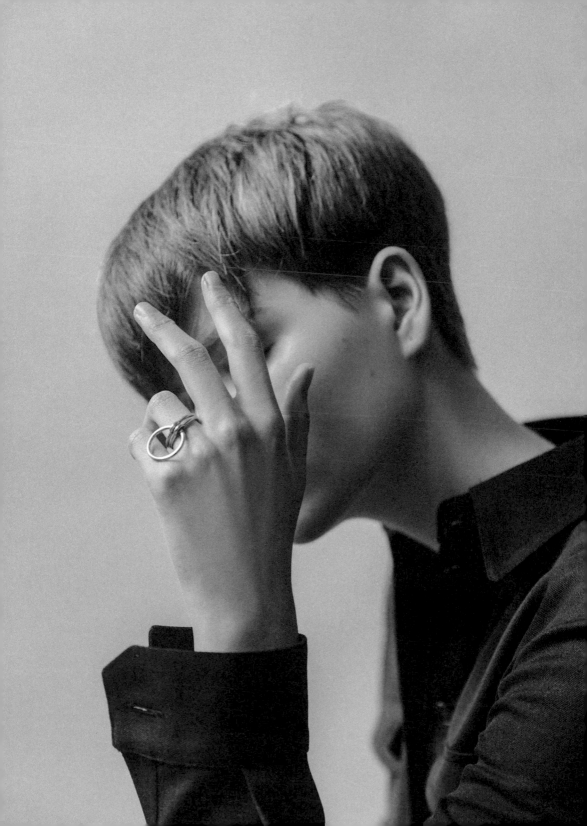

Shows are changing fast. The first show I ever did, over twenty years ago, was Preen by Thornton Bregazzi and since then I have gone on to head up shows for Jonathan Saunders, Michael van der Ham, Emilia Wickstead, Molly Goddard, Anya Hindmarch and Roksanda Ilincic to name just a few. There used to be this kind of mystique around the shows and the only way to see how a look really came to life was to actually be there and see it in action. Now you can be in your bedroom, anywhere in the world, and see the backstage happenings as soon as the first look has hit the catwalk. Fashion houses like Burberry stream the show live online and the backstage journalists share insights into how to create the looks and the products used in real time on social media. It's a far more inclusive process than it used to be. This is mostly great as it allows more people to get involved and get excited about fashion and hair and make-up, but I would be lying if I said I didn't miss some of that mystery.

Perhaps the most challenging thing that can happen to a hairdresser backstage is when a model is running exceptionally late from another show and when she arrives she has a tonne of product in her hair. When this happens you really can't throw your toys out of the pram, you just have to get her hair washed as fast as humanly possible so you can get her ready for the show. It's in stressful times like these that you count your lucky stars that your team are organised and on it. I have someone backstage at all times whose entire role is to keep track of who is late, who has arrived, who has had their hair done and who still needs to be seen. Without someone on top of that the whole process would descend into chaos.

There are some show hairdressers who are shouty and a bit irate – sadly I have seen a product thrown across the room more than once. It's undeniable that some hairdressers really get off on that kind of craziness but it's madness; there are already enough people screaming backstage before the show, and the hairdresser really doesn't need to join in too. And come on, let's be honest, it's just *hair!* It should be fun. I go out of my way to avoid that kind of frenetic atmosphere (and I would hope my team agree too!) and for me to be heard screaming backstage you would know that something close to catastrophic has happened. I like things to be calm and orderly and I feel the best shows are the ones where, of course, the hair looks incredible – but also when the team are working really well together and there's no drama. Even when you get thrown five girls to get ready ten minutes before the show, if everyone remains calm and pulls their weight you'll get through unscathed. You just don't need any more divas backstage, there are enough of them already.

I'm usually on a high after a show, and drowning in adrenaline, so I walk. Those three or four hours backstage can be incredibly intense and all the while you're engaged and focused to make sure everything is just right. It's a bit of an assault on the senses. So, for thirty or forty minutes after a show I just walk to take some time to myself and decompress. But despite the chaos there is still – after all these years of working on shows – nothing like seeing twenty or thirty girls all wearing the designer's collection, standing ready to walk onto that catwalk. When everything comes together it is just magic.

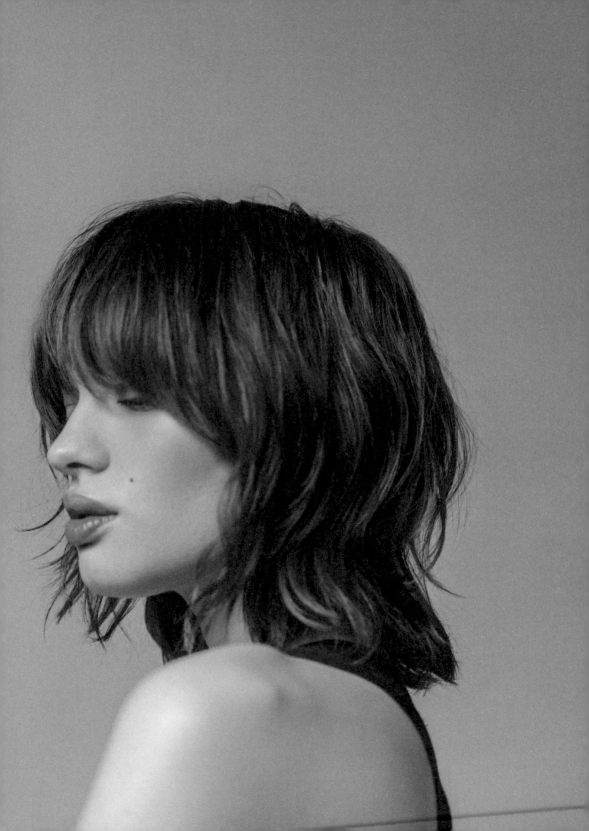

FIVE
LOOKS
THAT
ALWAYS
WORK

'The hair
equivalent of a
capsule wardrobe:
reliable, flattering
and always
appropriate'

My time backstage has shown me that some styles work on absolutely everyone every single time. Everyone loves to experiment with new styles and while that's to be commended, 99 per cent of the time it does pay to have a few staples in the bag that you *know* always look good and will see you through any situation whether that's an important meeting or a date. Think of these five looks as the hair equivalent of a capsule wardrobe: reliable, flattering and always appropriate. The best part? You don't have to be a hairdresser to pull them off.

THE CLASSIC

The classic is like a crisp white shirt that fits you perfectly. It's timeless; glossy and polished with a side parting and a touch of a wave that's universally flattering.

You need: Styling cream, a decent hairdryer with a nozzle attachment, a medium-sized round-barrelled ceramic brush and hairspray.

Step 1: Rub a 50p-sized blob of Almost Everything Cream between your hands to distribute the product and then work it through the mid-lengths to ends of your hair while it is still damp. This will add some heat protection, tame frizz and make your blow dry really last.

Step 2: Put your hair into a side parting and rough-dry it with just your hands and your hairdryer until it is about 95 per cent dry. You don't need to use the nozzle attachment yet and do not be tempted to touch a brush at this stage. Use your hands to drag the hair in a downwards direction to reduce any natural curl or frizz.

Step 3: Snap the nozzle onto your hairdryer and section out an area at the front of your hair that's roughly three inches wide and an inch deep.

Step 4: Wrap the section of hair around your round-barrelled brush and direct the airflow from your hairdryer directly at it from above. Gradually pull the brush down the length of hair in front of your face, allowing the hair to just smooth out and roll off the brush.

Step 5: Once you have completely dried the front, divide the rest of your hair into two sides from the crown down to the nape of your neck. Now just repeat the drying process around your head in sections about three inches wide.

Step 6: While blow-drying your top sections of hair, aim the hairdryer underneath your brush when it is close to your roots, which will give you plenty of lift. It seems fiddly at first but I promise you, with a little practice you'll be an expert.

Step 7: Finish with a light misting of hairspray.

Tip: Be patient with your hairdryer. Take your time running it down each section and you should find that you won't need to keep going over the same areas.

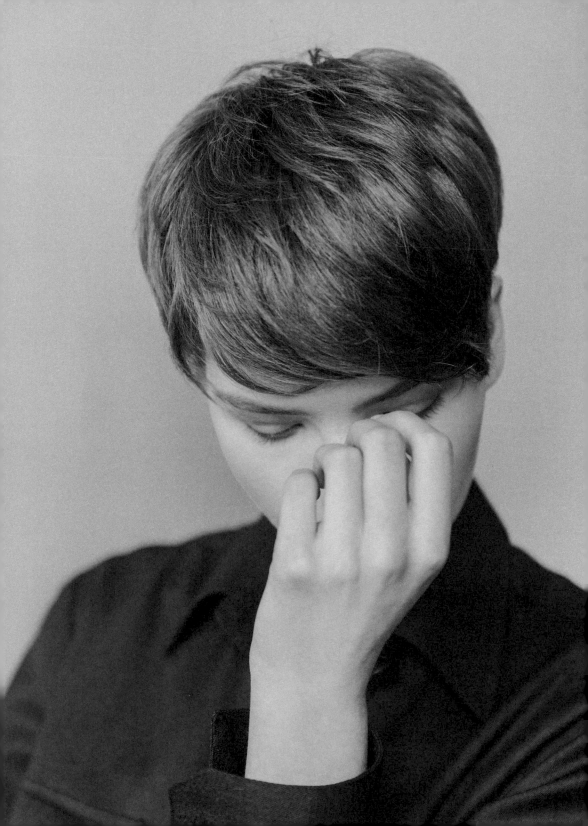

SMOOTH WAVY

This is a super-glamorous but understated style that somehow still manages to look quite effortless.

You need: A flat mixed-bristle brush, styling cream, a medium-sized curling tong with a clamp and hairspray.

Step 1: Use your mixed-bristle brush to remove any tangles and then apply a small amount of styling cream containing heat protector through dry hair.

Step 2: Divide your hair into two sections from your crown down to the nape of your neck.

Step 3: In sections begin tonging your hair. Keep the roots out of your tong and make sure you place the tong on top of your section and wrap it from underneath; this will give the right shape for this look. Slightly twist the hair as you wrap it around the barrel to intensify the wave before you clamp it.

Step 4: Leave the ends out of the barrel – you don't have to worry about getting it all in.

Step 5: Allow the hair to 'cook' around the barrel for about five seconds. If your hair is coloured or bleached it is going to grab the heat quickly, whereas if you have fewer layers and no colour it will take longer. As you remove the tong from the hair, catch the curl and let it lie in your hand for a few seconds to cool before you release it; this will give you a slightly tighter curl.

Step 6: Work your way around your entire head and when you have tonged the front sections tuck them behind your ears to allow them to cool.

Step 7: At this stage your hair will look very curly but it won't for long. Rub a touch more styling cream between your hands and comb your hands through your hair.

Step 8: Once your curls have cooled, *lightly* brush through them with your flat brush to soften the curls into waves. Finish with a mist of hairspray.

Tip: If your hair is on the fine side, lightly back-brush the underneath to create more volume.

WAVY GRAVY

We launched Wavy Gravy way back in 2002 and it still remains hugely popular in our blow dry bars, and for good reason. It's eternally cool and it's so laid-back it looks as though you've just got out of bed. Think tousled beach babe meets rock 'n' roll.

You need: A flat mixed-bristle brush, styling cream, a medium-sized curling tong and hairspray.

Step 1: Take your mixed-bristle brush through dry hair to remove any knots that might be lurking in there.

Step 2: Work a little heat protecting styling cream through your hair.

Step 3: Now, to tong. This is probably the simplest look involving tonging because you can be very random with your sections. Zero precision required. Put the barrel of the tong on top of your section and again twist the hair as you wrap it around. Leave the roots and the ends out so the finished look is more relaxed.

Step 4: Leave the hair around the barrel for just a matter of seconds, and then let it out. You don't need to allow the curl to cool in your hand because we're after a very loose wave. Work away around your head in no particular order.

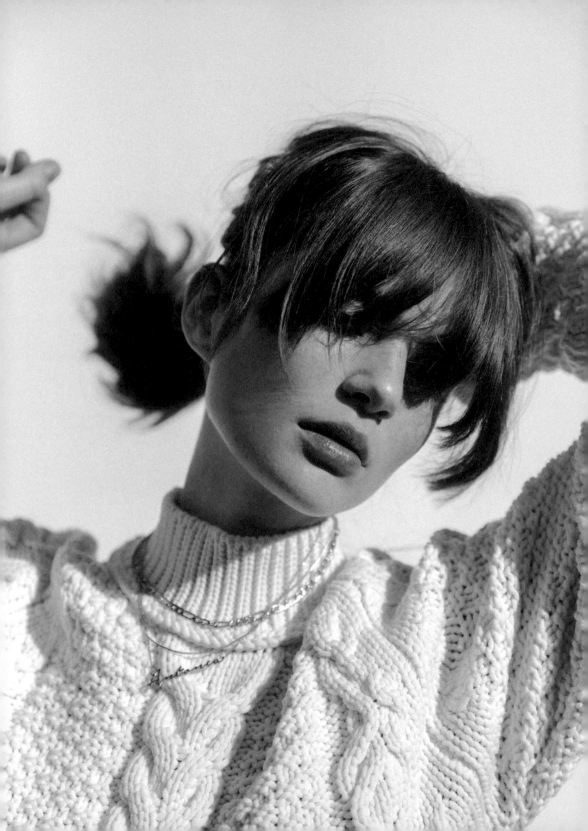

Step 5: When you get to your front sections, tuck your hair behind your ears as it sets to create a soft wave to frame your face.

Step 6: Once you have finished tonging just use your hands to rub sections of your hair between your palms to bring out a lived-in look.

Step 7: If you need it, use a little hairspray to set the waves.

Tip: Using a mirror can actually get you in a muddle as your reflection tells you to go one way while your brain sends you in the other. Go by feel alone. If you have gone too curly, clamp your straightening irons on your hair in places just to soften them.

A PROPER PONY

A ponytail with never go out of fashion and it's just about the most versatile look going. Wearing it low and sleek looks really androgynous and polished while wearing it high and flippy looks fun and youthful. For an everyday, every-occasion ponytail aim for somewhere in the middle.

You need: Styling cream, mixed-bristle brush, hairband or hair elastic, hairpins, grosgrain ribbon (optional), straightening irons, a clean and dry toothbrush, and hairspray.

Step 1: Smooth some styling cream through dry hair to reduce frizz.

Step 2. Use a mixed-bristle brush to brush your hair back into a ponytail. Gather it in the middle of the back of your head and tie it off with either a sleek hairband or elastic.

Step 3: Use your thumb and forefinger to pinch and soften the hair around your hairline to ensure the look isn't too severe.

Step 4: Now you have a couple of choices: either take a small section of hair from your ponytail and wrap it around the hair elastic to hide it and secure in place with a hairpin, or create a bow around the base with a length of grosgrain ribbon.

Step 5: If you want your ponytail to be super-sleek, now is the time to run your hair straighteners over it. Use a clean toothbrush and a little Elnett to smooth down any troublesome flyaways or the back of a comb to smooth out ridges. Or if you want more of a mussed-up texture, smooth a small amount of styling cream between your hands and use them to rough the hair up in places.

Step 6: Set your ponytail for the day with a misting of hairspray.

Tip: The more hair in a ponytail, the richer and more luscious it looks so you may benefit from adding a clip-in if your hair is not particularly plentiful.

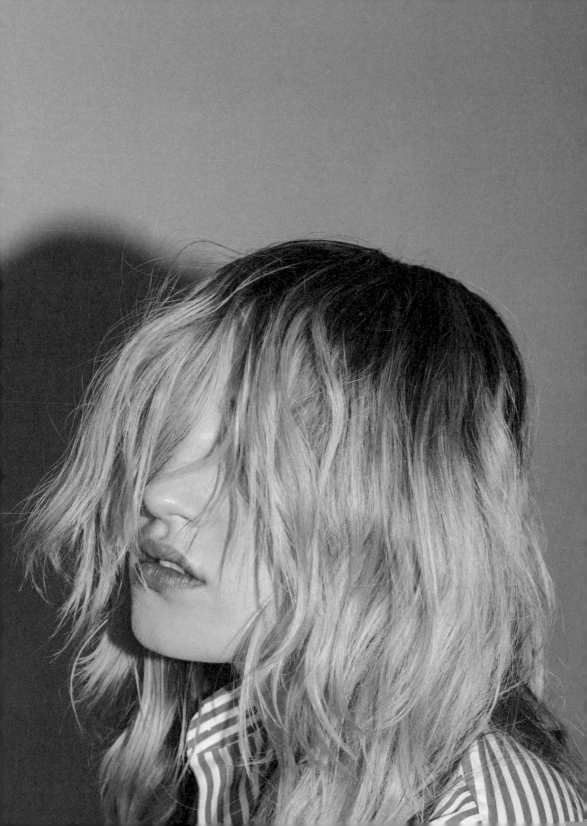

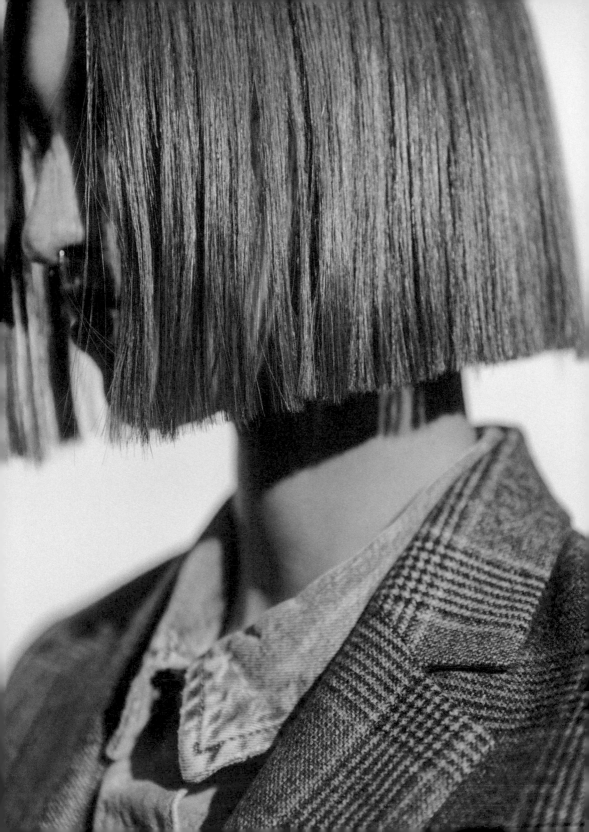

SUPER-STRAIGHT

Really, really straight hair looks very healthy and polished. It's the kind of hair that you can get to really shine and it looks so amazing when worn with a jersey Alice band.

You need: Styling cream, a comb, sectioning clips, a mixed-bristle brush, straightening irons and hairspray.

Step 1: Smooth a small amount of styling cream containing heat protection through completely dry hair. Use your hands like a comb to evenly distribute the cream throughout your hair. Heat protection is essential with this look as you're going to be using a lot of heat to get your hair poker straight.

Step 2: Decide on your parting and plot it in. There's something very sweet and naive about straight hair with a centre parting while a side parting will make the final result edgier and more graphic.

Step 3: For poker-straight hair you need to make sure all your strands look uniform, and the easiest way to do this is to section your hair and straighten one area at a time. I suggest brushing your hair through and then dividing it into four sections from your crown down to the nape of your neck and from ear to ear. Keep each section out of the way with a clip.

Step 4: Now straighten. Pass your iron down each section from roots to tips while simultaneously combing your hair. This will give you a very thorough and precise finish.

Step 5: Once you have finished straightening use a touch more styling cream to ramp up the shine and smooth any flyaways that have appeared around your hairline.

Tip: Straightening your hair naturally takes out some of the volume so you may want to add some clip-in hair extensions if you want bigger hair.

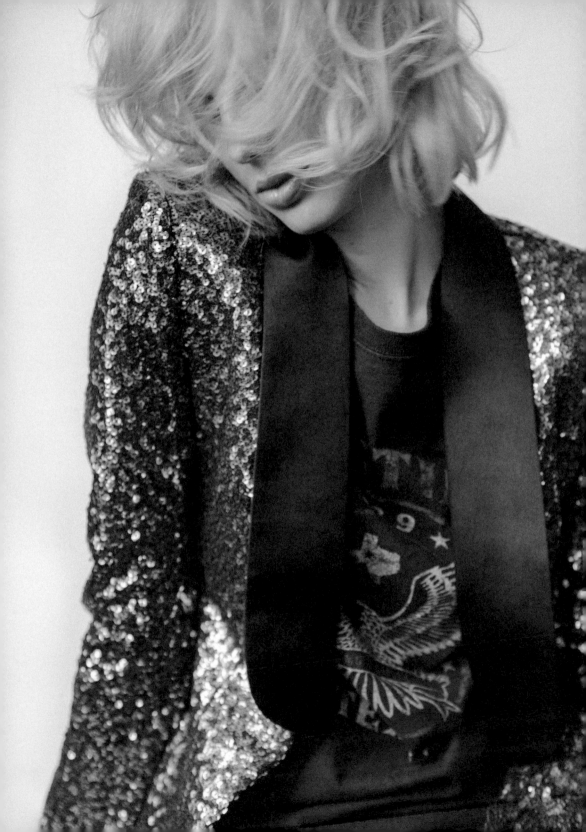

HAIR
AND
CLOTHES

'Do whatever you
want with your hair
so long as it makes
you feel good'

Hair can be the kick-off point or the finishing touch of your look. But your personal style is built on more than just your hair; the clothes you wear, how you apply your make-up, and even how you walk, all contribute in some degree to your overall image. I do believe that the clothes you wear and how you choose to style your hair should share some common ground. If your fashion sense could be described as easy and nonchalant then I wouldn't think that you would want to wear fussy and overly groomed hair, for example.

That said, I am opposed to the idea that what you wear should directly feed into how you style your hair. A look that is too matchy-matchy is never a good one in my opinion and I don't believe that there are prescribed hairstyles for certain clothes. In fact, it flies in the face of everything that I believe as a stylist. What one woman thinks of as the perfect style for an evening dress might seem completely mad to someone else. Hair should never be proscriptive. As far as I'm concerned, you should do whatever you want with your hair so long as it makes you feel good.

As a hairdresser I prefer to think of style – and how hair relates to fashion – more broadly. If I'm getting someone ready for a red-carpet event, for example, I will naturally look at the dress first but I won't be thinking, 'Okay, that's a full-length gown and so it requires a neat chignon.' That is just far too formulaic and lacking in imagination if you ask me.

The best way to decide on a hairstyle that complements what you are going to wear is to ask yourself whether your clothing could do with dialling up or dialling down. For example, if you have a formal dress in a bold block colour or which includes some statement-making details, perhaps an embellished neckline or embroidery, then use your hair to dial down the look and wear it simpler. In this instance a soft up-do would be great. If the clothes you are wearing are making a statement then it's important that your hair doesn't jar – *sometimes* the hair needs to take a back seat to the clothing.

If, however, you're wearing something simple – a tee perhaps, or a simpler, more understated dress – then use your hair to dial things up a little bit by adding more texture, more volume or maybe even a hair accessory in the form of an Alice band. Or go all out on a sleek and graphic style on a side parting. This is one of those occasions where you can let your hair do the talking and your clothes are the support act.

It's important that you always look like you, and never as though you're playing dress-up. Whether you're suited and booted for an important work meeting or popping to the pub to meet your friends for lunch, there should be something about your hair that speaks of your own personal style. If you're known for a cut like a bob or Antibob, play around with the texture; if you normally wear a ponytail, you can make it more polished and glossy with a bit of height when wearing a beautiful gown, or tie some ribbon around the base if you're wearing something more casual and want to add a touch of interest. If your hair is long and you always wear it down, you can easily dial up the drama by adding some waves if you have some-where special to be.

Your own style should work with anything you choose to wear – you just need to learn which bits you like to play up and play down. The idea that you should overhaul the way you look to fall in line with a specific event, or that your clothes should dictate how the rest of you looks, is completely ludicrous and more than a little outdated.

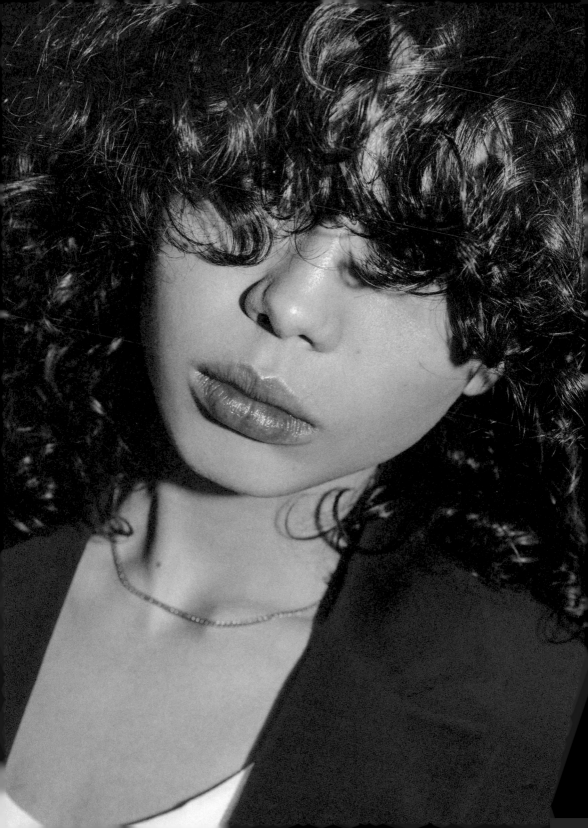

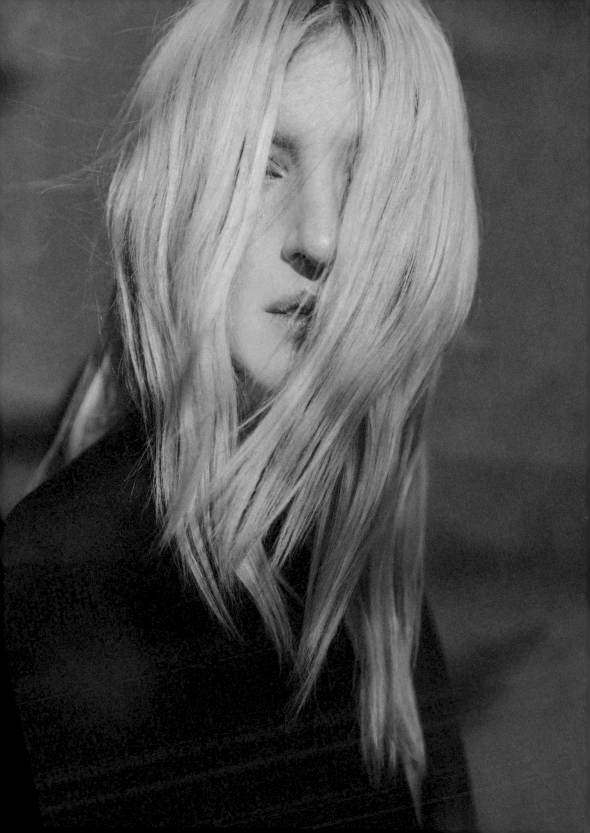

HAIR
ENHANCEMENTS

'After all,
hair should
be fun'

Back in the eighties my dad used to sell hair accessories at his salon. The entire front of his shop was dedicated to them. He sold just the most incredible pieces from the likes of Nina Ricci, Moschino and Alexandre de Paris. Women would come in all the time – even if they didn't have an appointment – and spend hundreds and hundreds of pounds on hair accessories.

The eighties really embraced hair adornments and it wasn't unusual for women of all ages to wear oversized ribbons and headbands; but this was the decade of excess and optimism, when anything truly felt possible.

Things quickly became quite serious after that and hair accessories were labelled immature and frivolous. I'm glad now that a little of this fun attitude is coming back into styling. After all, hair *should* be fun. Accessories and embellishments are a playful way of experimenting with how you look – with a bold headband or a clip-in hairpiece you can completely change your appearance without any kind of commitment whatsoever. Extensions, weaves, braids, 'winges', bands, accessories and scarves are great and inexpensive conduits of change.

There is no reason why you should feel silly wearing a hair accessory or while enhancing your natural hair with more of it. There is no rule that says you can't experiment and be playful with your hair – thank heavens. Sure, some accessories (like the bows made of hair that were everywhere a couple of years ago) are a flash in the pan or really only appropriate at a specific moment in time but some, like the Alice band and the intricate clips, slides and barrettes at Simone Rocha, are never *not* great. Even the scrunchie is making a defiant comeback despite the odds; I know some people hate them but they're playful and a fun way of channelling an eighties moment.

Enhancing and embellishing your hair is one of the few areas of your appearance where you can afford to be completely frivolous. So what if the bow you're wearing today looks outdated tomorrow? Who cares if you have hair extensions down to your behind when a shoulder-skimming length is currently in vogue? I am completely behind the notion of playing dress-up with hair but there is, of course, a fine line between elegantly embellished and looking like a part-time Vegas showgirl.

ACCESSORIES

Despite the stellar success my dad had selling pricey designer hair accessories in the eighties, I don't think it's worth spending a lot of cash on them now. The high street is a treasure chest of beautiful and affordable accessories. In fact, at one point we were thinking about selling hair accessories at Hershesons and then we thought, really what's the point? The high street already has this sewn up and it's inherently good at offering up inexpensive, fun and playful accessories, with & Other Stories and H&M the best of a good bunch.

Unless you're buying an accessory for a special occasion such as your wedding – where you'll likely keep it a lifetime – I think spending vast sums of money on an accessory that may well look completely past its prime in less than a year is a waste. My thinking is that diamante is never okay, as it will always look a bit cheap. The only exception is if it's Chanel, because I firmly believe that Chanel anything is nothing but chic.

Another favourite accessory of mine is the Syd Pin. This chic and versatile hairpin was created by hairstylist and great friend Syd Hayes when he was working on a Fashion Week show. It sums up everything a great hair accessory should be: easy to use and beautiful.

Hair accessories can be quite seasonal and what feels right in this moment might be a different story altogether in a couple of years. However, there are some styles that *always* feel right. It's also important to consider your outfit and how you're wearing your hair when you're thinking about what to put in it.

Hair accessories tend to look best when teamed with an uncomplicated hairstyle: a simple half-up or sleek ponytail. When worn with an elaborate hairstyle, it can all start to look a little too much. The same rule applies with your clothes. Outrageously embellished and intricate clothing is best left to do all the talking; it doesn't need another force vying for attention. Hair accessories look utterly stunning when worn with minimalistic hair. A Céline-esque barrette wouldn't look out of place in even the most corporate of environments. Thanks to Céline, we're now spoilt for choice when it comes to elegantly simple, and affordable-ish, metal hair barrettes, as the high street and some higher-end stores have scrambled to produce their own take on this catwalk favourite.

Offcuts of fabric and lengths of material are quite useful so I suggest familiarising yourself with your local haberdashery. I like to use strips of jersey fabric to fashion my own DIY headbands, while grosgrain ribbon and leather cord look really great tied around hair. The shop VV Rouleaux is a brilliant resource for ribbons, cords and fabrics, and somewhat of a must-visit destination for designers, stylists and anyone working in the creative industries. My backstage kit is usually overflowing with various pieces of fabric and I have created some of my favourite Fashion Week looks with them. Roksanda Ilinčić is a designer who really enjoys hair accessories and I have created a few for her shows; one time we used neoprene to fashion some hair bows and another time we came up with a grosgrain-ribbon headband. Accessories give you a look without having to do too much work to your hair; you can actually get away with really underplaying your hair when you're wearing a fabulous accessory because that's what becomes the talking point.

EXTENSIONS

I really only use extensions for adding volume rather than length. They're fine if you just want to bump up your length by a couple of inches but I really don't think that they should be used to take your hair from short to long. As far as I'm concerned, they just don't look entirely convincing when used that way.

Used properly, however, they are just brilliant. If your hair is thinning slightly, then you will find a couple of rows of clip-in extensions totally revolutionary. If you need a little more length, and something longer-lasting, then you can achieve beautiful, thick, luscious locks with some permanently bonded extensions. There are so many choices now, both of the temporary and permanent kind, that there is an option for everyone.

CLIP-INS

Unless you have a huge amount of hair already, most women can benefit from a little extra volume and thickness – perhaps not every day (though there is no reason why not) but certainly for an evening out or a special occasion. I recommend keeping a few rows of clip-in extensions in your hair wardrobe to add into your hair when you're creating a look that requires some more volume. If your hair is usually reluctant to hold a curl or a wave, popping in a few wefts can really help. Our clip-in extensions – while made of human hair – are processed so that they can hold the shape created by heated styling tools for longer without dropping out. By placing a few wefts around your head and tonging everything, even if the style falls out of your natural hair, your clip-in hair will remain in good shape.

There's a bit of a misconception around clip-in hair; many stylists will tell you to either match it to your own hair colour, or dye it the same colour you dye your own. I suggest that rather than matching, buy a shade ever so slightly lighter or darker than your natural colouring to give the illusion of more depth and even more hair. When your hair is all one colour it can look very solid and a little outdated. At Hershesons, our range consists of ten to twelve shades but we're adding some balayage options into the mix, which have a marginally darker root area and lighter ends. Clip-ins vary dramatically in price but, as with anything, the better the quality the more they are likely to cost; as a very loose idea you're looking at around £80 to £150 depending on the amount of hair and the length.

There was a time when women were squeamish about wearing hair enhancements made from real human hair, and nine times out of ten they would steer towards a synthetic option. Real hair offers so many benefits that you don't get with the synthetic kind; you can use styling tools on

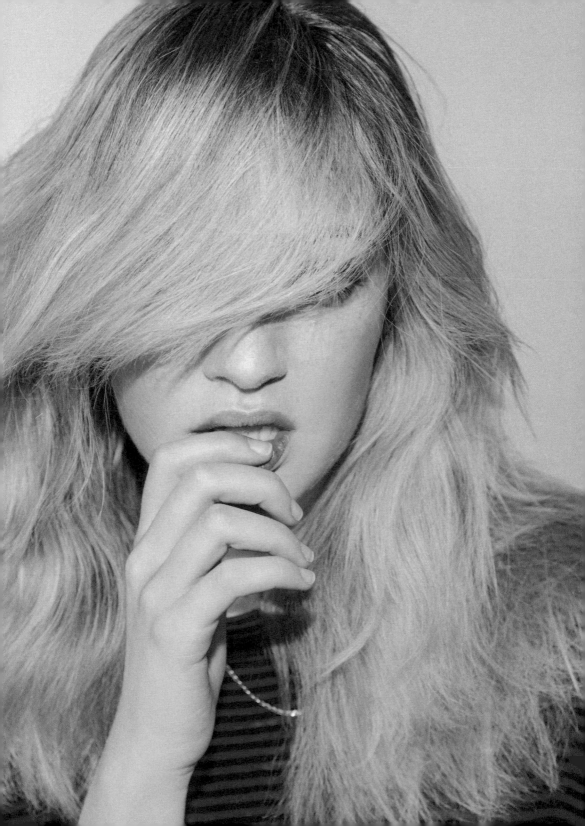

them for one – which means that you can wear them straight, wavy or curly and not be limited to one style – you can wash and dry them in the same way that you do your normal hair and with the same products, and they feel and look far more convincing. Thankfully this is something women are recognising now and so synthetic hair is largely on the out.

FILLERS

Extensions are far more bespoke now and less one-size-fits-all. Fillers are a relatively new idea for most women but they are brilliant when you're experiencing some thinning in places. Rather than a full head of extensions, fillers are placed just where you need some more density to give you the illusion of a thicker hairline. They are extremely tiny bonds, which are placed very close to the scalp and around where you would typically lose hair as you get older, and instead of glue, the bonds are fixed in place with heat alone. If you take care of them they'll last for up to three months, at which point you need to come back into the salon to have them taken out. Fillers are something that we have done at Hershesons for a while now but I am sure there are other salons out there doing something similar so ask around; if your hairdresser doesn't do it then ask them to suggest someone who does. The more people who request these kinds of treatments, the more salons will start investing in them. They cost somewhere around £250, but again this price could go up or down depending on where the salon is, the quality of the hair they're using and how much you're having applied.

TAPES / SANDWICHES

Tapes are the exciting new kid on the block; they're basically a strip of hair that gets slotted amongst your own. One strip lies flat on top of a section of hair, while another strip lies directly underneath – effectively you're sandwiching sections of your real hair in between strips of fake. They lie super-flat and there is no glue or clips, which makes them pretty much invisible to the eye. At around £70 they're on the affordable side of hair extensions and the best bit is that they are reusable. When you're ready to have them taken out, your stylist will remove them and have them cleaned ready to use again.

PERMANENT HAIR EXTENSIONS

A full head of permanent extensions is eternally popular with clients and it's likely to remain that way for some time. They can be expensive, but they provide long-lasting extra length, volume and density without the faff of putting in and taking out clip-ins every day. Still, I think even permanent extensions are best only for enhancing your own hair, when you're filling and thickening or maybe adding one or two inches in length. When you use extensions to lengthen your hair from, say, just below your collarbone right down your back, you're really asking for trouble. They are really tricky to pull off and will never look entirely convincing. The price can be upwards of £500 but the quality of the hair, the experience and reputation of the salon, the length and how much you're having will determine the price. Most salons insist on a consultation first (and if *they* don't, *you* should) and it's then that you will find out the exact cost. Many salons now do permanent hair extensions but it's really important that you ask to see their before and after shots; some salons will post images of their clients' hair to their social media accounts so be sure to check those too.

Great Lengths is probably the most globally known maker of hair extensions and they work with over 30,000 salons around the world so most cities should have a salon or two that uses them – you can check their website for a full list.

Extensions are best worn for at least a few months before having them taken out as your stylist will often have to cut into your own hair a little to help blend them with your new hair. If your extensions come out too early, and your own hair hasn't had much of an opportunity to grow, you may find that you'll end up with hair that's slightly shorter than it was to begin with.

As with anything, the difference between brilliantly convincing extensions and extensions that look absolutely horrendous is down to the skill of the stylist and not just the quality of the hair you're using. A great stylist will often cut the bonds into smaller pieces so they're less detectable and so they can be really precise with where they are adding volume – this is as much of an art form as colouring or cutting. Some of the best hair-extension professionals are colourists too because they understand how the hair blends.

If you're in the market for hair extensions you may find the options and terminology a little baffling. I'm hoping to make it easier for you:

Remy Hair is human hair that has been collected in a particular way so that all the hair cuticles fall in one direction and are less likely to matt and tangle. It's from a single donor and has been minimally processed so it's likely to be quite expensive and only used in good-quality extensions. There are a lot of companies on the internet who claim their hair extensions are Remy when they are not. If you find that the hair mats and knots it will most likely not be Remy. If the price looks too good to be true, it probably is as they are likely to be mixing natural and synthetic hair in one bundle. I would be careful where you get your hair from; go on recommendations when you can and always look for reviews.

Non-Remy Hair is probably the most widely available human hair. The roots and tips are mixed up so the cuticles do not all lie in one direction and the hair has been chemically processed.

Virgin Hair is donated human hair from one donor that hasn't been chemically processed in any way. Virgin hair is carefully acquired from hair merchants and will be Remy.

Single Drawn Hair is made up of 50 per cent full-length hair and 50 per cent mixed-length hair. These kinds of extensions often look more natural as they mimic the variety seen in your own hair. However, if you're looking for impossibly thick, glamorous, big hair you're unlikely to achieve that with Single Drawn Hair. Single Drawn Hair responds better to heat so it's a good option if you like to create a more lived-in look with tongs.

Double Drawn Hair is made up of 70 to 80 per cent full-length hairs and a much smaller percentage of varying lengths. There's more hair involved so naturally it's more expensive and it delivers big, voluminous hair. Double Drawn Hair tends to be more expensive because it's *technically* perfect hair, which is great if you want one big glossy mane of hair. But, if you want more guts and body and you want to tong it, Double Drawn Hair really is not ideal because it's too heavy. In this instance, the more affordable Single Drawn Hair is far more appropriate.

THE WINGE

A full, perfectly positioned fringe looks chic. Full stop. However, they can be tricky to style if you have a cowlick or a wave to your hair, a nightmare to maintain if you're prone to frizz, and they require commitment as they need trimming far more often than the rest of your hair. If you have toyed with the idea of a fringe but you're not sold on the amount of work that goes into one, then you really ought to get a clip-in fringe, or a Winge (a wig/fringe) as they are known. They cost around £30 and instantly add drama to your look; they're already styled to lie perfectly and they're commitment-free as you can simply remove them at the end of the day.

Smooth your own hair away from your face and tuck it behind your ears if you can to keep it out of the way. Each Winge comes with three clips; open up the clips and place the fringe into your hair with the middle pointy section nestled back towards your crown. Snap the clips in place and bring the rest of your hair forward again.

I suggest that rather than spending an inordinate amount of time trying to convincingly blend your faux fringe with the rest of your hair, simply pair it with a wide Alice band to hide the seam.

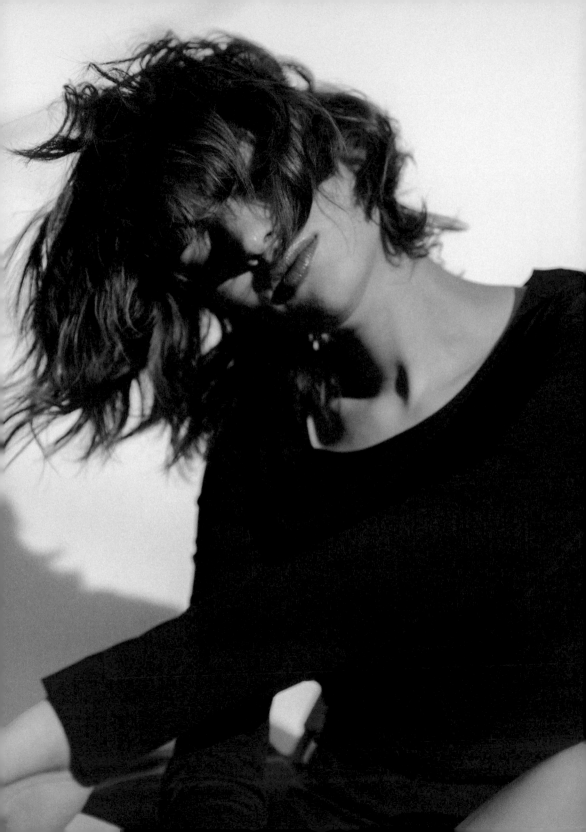

LET'S TALK ABOUT SEX

'Sexiness comes down to attitude; own what makes you unique and love your hair'

Hair is inherently sexy – sometimes, in fact, it can be positively filthy. Just by repositioning your ponytail you can take your hair from preppy to provocative, the right kind of waves look as though they have been raked through in a moment of lust, and an up-do that hints of restraint sends an entirely different message when it is a little mussed up and 'undone' in places.

Care to admit it or not, it is human nature to give a shit about what others think of the way you look – *especially* if it's a person who you fancy. Everything you do and say and every gesture that you make is sending a subtle – or in some cases, not-so-subtle – cue to the object of your desires. And there's absolutely nothing wrong with that – you can be smart, successful, independent *and* desirable.

That said, there is no hard-and-fast rule as to what the opposite sex – or indeed the same sex – will interpret as sexy hair (if there was, and I knew it, I would be a very rich man). To make use of a tired cliché: just as beauty is in the eye of the beholder, so too is sexiness. I have a friend, for example, who thinks that fringes are the most disgusting things ever and could never fancy a girl with one, whereas there are countless examples of super-sexy fringes like Uma Thurman in *Pulp Fiction* or Brigitte Bardot. One person's turn-on can just as easily be another's turn-off but, I suppose, that's what keeps things interesting.

Here are my thoughts on sexy hair:

Sexy hair does not necessarily mean long hair. I repeat, hair does not have to be long to be sexy. I hate the assumption that in order for hair to be sexy it has to be long; in fact, I find it quite offensive. Think of a nineties Winona Ryder with short hair, Gwyneth Paltrow in *Sliding Doors*, Demi Moore in *Ghost*, Linda Evangelista's cropped hair in a series of Peter Lindbergh photographs from the late eighties, and Natalie Portman in *Closer* (or let's be honest, Natalie Portman in anything) – these are short hairstyles that are surely undeniably sexy by anyone's standards.

That's not to say long hair can't also be incredibly sexy. Two words: Kate and Gisele. Need I say more? Thought not.

There's a lot to be said for changing up your parting. I think partings say a lot about your character. A centre parting looks cute but on very curly hair it can, at times, appear a little downbeat. Moving your parting a centimetre or so to one side changes everything; suddenly you look more carefree and flirtatious. Switching up your parting really changes the message you're putting out there so play around with its positioning.

Small changes can be just as, if not more, impactful than the bigger ones. It's not always about cutting your hair off. A tweak to your colour, adding some layers to encourage more natural movement or slicking down your side parting to give your hair a very luxe, boyish, old Armani feel can be just as powerful and make just as much of a statement as cutting your hair shorter.

What men and women find sexy is wildly subjective. Remember, what might be unappealing to one person might be sexy as hell for another. Who is to say what is alluring or intriguing or memorable? These things mean different things to different people. Never be shy or embarrassed about any little quirks in your hair; play them up and embrace them because I can guarantee you, there are people out there who will love them.

Confidence is oh so sexy. In my opinion, sexiness comes down to attitude, so you should own what makes you unique and love your hair. You can have the perfect cut and an immaculate blow dry but if you're not comfortable in your own skin you are not going to feel sexy. Feeling sexy is just as important, if not more, than looking sexy. Wear your hair however the hell you want – just feel assured and confident with it. Sexy hair is a bit like a sexy dress: for it to feel natural and authentic you have to wear the hair, not the other way around.

Sexy hair is touchable hair. Hair that looks hard and sticky is not sexy. You want the person you desire to fantasise about running their fingers through your hair and that's not so easy to do when it looks as though it could

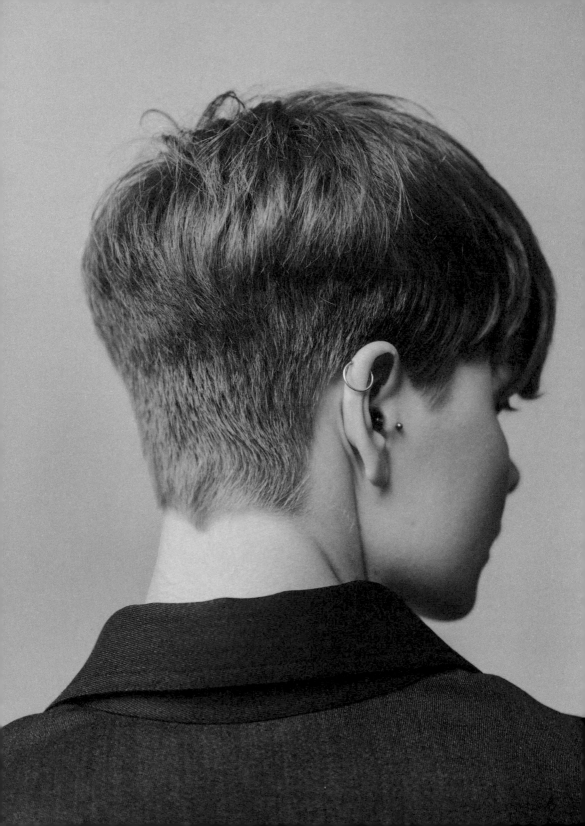

withstand an earthquake. If you're going on a date or banking on a night of fun between the sheets, ease up on the hairspray.

To some extent, sexy hair is all about make-believe. Sexy hair is a little like no-make-up make-up: a whole lot of trickery and consideration goes into a look that's ultimately meant to appear as though very little has been done to it. Whether we're talking about a first date, or taking the perfect picture for your Tinder or online dating profile, you want to convince the onlooker that your impossibly sexy hair is something you were born with, even if it took an hour with a curling wand to achieve.

Never cut your hair when you're angry. I know it's tempting after a devastating breakup to book into the first salon you lay eyes on and get a chop – a fresh start is so desperately needed when you go through something traumatic. But please, never ever – ever – get a dramatic cut when you're angry. A haircut is not a viable tool of revenge (there are far more creative ways of getting even) and the only person likely to regret your decision in the long term is you. The only exception is if you genuinely want a change and you're approaching the decision with enthusiasm.

Sexy hair should never look contrived. I think there is one overriding factor about sexy hair and that's if it ever feels too manicured or too worked, or the hand of a hairdresser has been in it for too long, I can guarantee you that your hair is about as far from sexy as you can get. Dial it back a lot.

Keep it clean. Your love life doesn't have to be clean but your hair *should*. There is nothing sexier than the smell of someone's hair. If your partner is taller than you, remember that the top of your head is likely nestled under their nose quite a lot so make the moment pleasurable with clean scalp and hair.

Scent can ramp up the sex factor. 'Fragrance layering' is industry jargon for wearing multiple scents. In most cases I think it's just another ruse to get women to buy more perfume, but there is definitely something to be said for subtly fragrancing your hair (subtly being the operative word here).

Just think about it: your date leans in for a kiss or a hug and they can't help but inhale the scent of your hair, it's intoxicating. Every time you move the delicious scent of your hair will surreptitiously waft in his or her direction and, if the night heats up, as your skin flushes and the temperature of your scalp warms up, the fragrance will deepen and intensify. If that isn't erotic I don't know what is.

Tempted? Try these fail-safe hair fragrances (you can, of course, use normal perfume but they tend to contain more alcohol than their hair-friendly counterparts and may make your hair feel dry and dehydrated):

Frederic Malle Carnal Flower Hair Mist contains a hefty dose of tuberose – a white flower that the Victorians actually kept from young woman for fear that one whiff might incite them to spontaneously combust into an orgasm. I'm not kidding. Tuberose smells like sex so handle with care.

Tom Ford Black Orchid Hair Mist is dark and a little twisted with black truffle, fresh bergamot, blackcurrant, black orchid (of course) and fruit accords. The original *parfum* is quite addictive, and this is too. This mist also has a shot of vitamin B5 so you're simultaneously conditioning your hair.

Byredo Gypsy Water Hair Perfume is assertive and confidence-boosting and ideal for a first date. It's laden with bergamot, pepper, incense and orris. There's also an undercurrent of steamy amber, sandalwood and vanilla, which are traditionally warm and sexy smells.

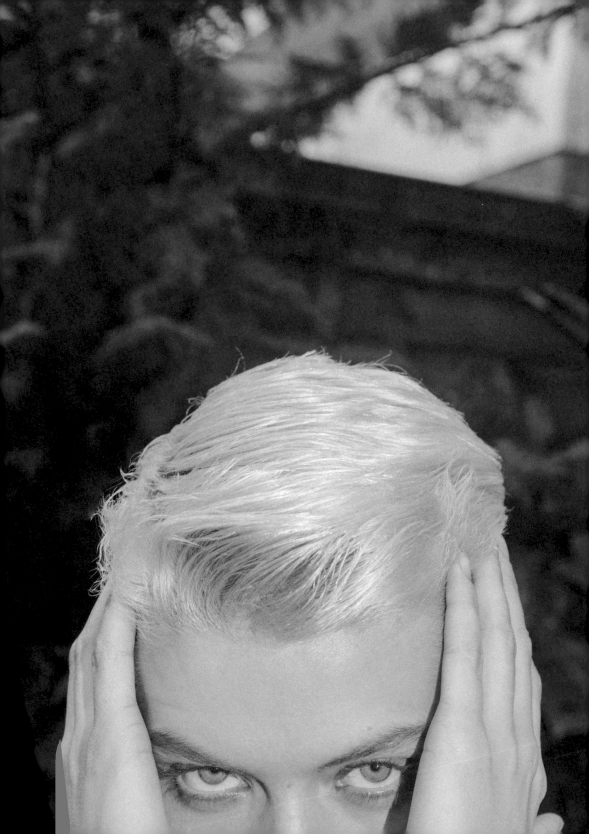

GREAT HAIR FROM THE INSIDE OUT

'Enjoy the
best hair of
your life'

To have truly great hair you have to think beyond the styling products and heated tools that you're using – a more 360-degree holistic approach is in order if you want to enjoy the best hair of your life. Your lifestyle, what you eat, the supplements you take and your stress levels all have a say in how your hair looks, feels and grows.

DIET

Most diets – even the so-called healthy ones – do not include the right mix and quantities of nutrients needed in order to grow great hair. Sure, your diet might be bursting at the seams with fruits and vegetables but this does little good for your hair if you are not consuming enough protein and calories. Hair cells are the second-fastest-growing cells in the human body – that's pretty prolific behaviour for something most people consider to be dead. Around 85 to 90 per cent of the hair on your head is in its growth phase at any one time and each and every one of those hairs require a lot of energy to thrive.

Hair is not a vital organ or tissue – you can quite easily live without it – and so when your body is run-down or ill it will channel all of its energies to where it is needed the most. Ultimately – as much as we love it – hair *is* expendable and your body will ruthlessly ignore its nutrient needs if there is anything more vital that demands its attention. This makes hair a fairly accurate barometer of someone's health. In fact, by studying a single strand of hair up close under a microscope to see where it thins, a trichologist can usually get a very good indication of your health and stress levels over the years, or however long that strand has been rooted in your scalp. Hair and scalp problems can arise from too little of certain nutrients in your diet and, in some cases, a poor diet alone can be responsible for hair loss. Hair cells need a good balance of proteins, complex carbohydrates, vitamins and minerals to perform properly and any diet that excludes even one vital food group is a poor one for your hair.

I must caution you that a certain amount of patience is required when making hair-friendly dietary changes as it will take *at least* three months before your efforts become visible.

PROTEIN

If you notice that your hair never grows past a certain point then it could be that you're eating insufficient amounts of protein. 80 to 85 per cent of hair is made up of a specific protein called keratin; this is what gives hair its strength, resilience and flexibility. Including a good amount of protein in your diet will ensure that your hair remains in its anagen, or growth, phase for as long as possible, otherwise it tends to become weak and brittle and snap before it has reached its full potential.

However, not all protein is equal as far as hair is concerned; primary proteins – which are animal proteins including eggs, fish, lean and red meat and poultry – are the very best kind for your hair because the body easily makes good use of their amino acids. Egg whites, in particular, are thought to be an excellent source of protein for the body. Of course, not everyone can, or wants, to eat animal products, in which case you should fill up on beans, lentils, nuts, tofu and pulses – they don't contain as many amino acids as animal proteins but they are not to be sniffed at either.

Breakfast and lunch are good times to meet your protein quota for the day. Breakfast is an especially good time as it's the first shot of energy to your body after its fast while you were sleeping. Trichologists and dieticians suggest eating around 120 grams of protein with breakfast and lunch.

IRON

Iron deficiency is the guilty culprit behind many instances of hair loss. Gorgeous, lustrous hair and a healthy and balanced scalp demand a nutrient-rich blood supply. If your iron levels are low and you have become anaemic, your scalp and its follicles will not be getting what they need and as a result your hair's growth cycle can go haywire. This means that you may notice more hair falling out when you wash and brush it.

If your levels of iron are low enough to impact your health and hair growth you may notice some fatigue, headaches, shortness of breath, dizziness, paleness, insomnia and a difficulty concentrating. In every instance your first port of call should be a GP or health practitioner for a simple blood test. Most of the time an iron deficiency can be rectified by a few dietary tweaks, but occasionally your doctor may suggest taking iron tablets to help move the process along.

The best, and most bio-available (meaning easily used by the body) sources of iron can be found in animal products such as fish, chicken and red meat. But don't forget your veggies: spinach, broccoli, kale and other leafy green vegetables, plus legumes including lentils, beans and peas, are great sources of iron too. Iron does, however, have a little quirk; it can only be properly absorbed into the bloodstream if it is eaten alongside vitamin C, which is why vegetables like broccoli and spinach are so valuable as they contain both iron *and* vitamin C. Alternatively, follow your iron-rich meal with a piece of citrus fruit, or add lemon juice to your meat and greens.

VITAMIN A

If your scalp is itchy and easily irritated try upping the amount of vitamin A you are consuming in your diet. Your body uses vitamin A to create sebum, the oily substance that keeps your skin soft and your scalp well-moisturised. Without sebum your scalp can become dry, flaky, tight and uncomfortable (not to mention your skin becomes dehydrated and lines and wrinkles more prominent). Some animal products, including beef liver, contain vitamin A but your best sources are yellow and orange vegetables like carrots, peppers, squashes and sweet potatoes. You will also find some in spinach, kale, greens, broccoli and bok choy.

VITAMIN C

The powerful antioxidant, vitamin C, plays a vital role in the creation of collagen. You're likely already familiar with collagen when it comes to your skincare routine where it plumps up and strengthens cells and gives skin a smooth and cushioned feel. Collagen serves a very similar purpose for hair; it provides strength and flexibility, boosts iron absorption and – thanks to its antioxidant properties – it helps to neutralise harmful free radicals.

Vitamin C is what's known as an 'essential' vitamin as the human body – remarkable though it is – is unable to produce it on its own or even store it. This is why it is crucial – not just for your hair but for your overall health – to eat foods that are rich in vitamin C every single day. Without fail. No excuses. In addition to its hair-boosting abilities, vitamin C supports wound healing and maintains tissue and bone health. It really is that brilliant.

Of course, a vitamin C deficiency is likely to come about if you're not eating enough of the stuff, but indulging in too much alcohol, smoking and being ill will also deplete what vitamin C you do have in your body.

Vitamin C can be found in the obvious places like lemons, oranges, berries, kiwis, watermelon and sweet potatoes but you'll also find it in kale, broccoli and Brussels sprouts with the added bonus of a hefty dose of iron. Be conscious of the fact that – as a water-soluble vitamin – you lose vitamin C in the cooking process so try to eat your veggies as close to raw as possible.

VITAMIN D

Experts believe that the vast majority of people, regardless of where they live in the world, have a vitamin D deficiency. If you have a dark complexion your skin is so well protected from UV that your body has a hard time utilising it to create the vitamin. SPF30 – which is absolutely necessary to protect skin from developing potential melanomas and ageing prematurely – reduces vitamin D production in the skin by up to 97.5 per cent and many of us spend most of the daylight hours working indoors. That's bad news all round as vitamin D plays a part in everything from fertility to brain health and bone density to maintaining a healthy heart.

As far as hair goes, research suggests that vitamin D can help create new follicles and ultimately increase the number of hairs on your head. It is believed that vitamin D reanimates dormant follicles and pushes them into a growth phase. It's far from a cure for baldness but it is definitely a step in the right direction. Vitamin D can be found in leafy greens like spinach, kale and collard greens, in egg yolks and some vitamin-D-fortified dairy products, breads and pasta. Vitamin D is also great in supplement form as you would really have to take an awful lot to get anywhere near toxicity (more on that later in the chapter).

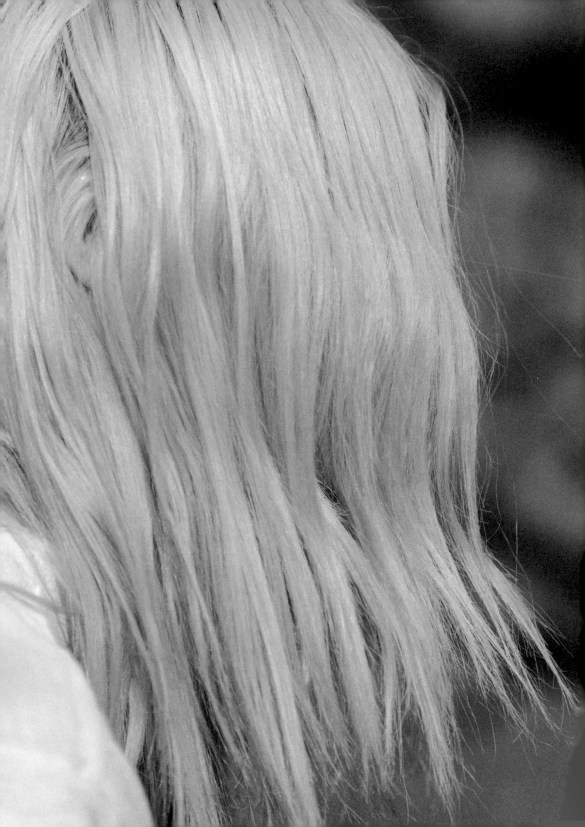

VITAMIN E

Vitamin E is a bit of an over-achiever; it prevents dry and brittle hair, helps to keep your scalp well-moisturised *and* it supports the growth of capillaries, which boost blood flow to your hair follicles, stimulating growth and maintaining hair health. It's also a stellar antioxidant and so helps fend off damage caused by free radicals. If ever there was a teacher's pet of the vitamin world it's vitamin E.

Incorporate almonds, spinach, sweet potatoes, avocados, sunflower seeds and olive oil into your daily diet to ensure a bountiful supply of the good stuff.

HEALTHY FATS

Since the eighties, 'fat' has been unfairly tarnished as a dirty word but in truth, not all fats are made equal. Some fats – particularly non-saturated ones like polyunsaturated and monounsaturated fats – are absolutely essential for good health and great hair and skin. Saturated fats are not so bad if they're only enjoyed from time to time, and trans fats – such as those found in fast foods like crisps and ready meals – are downright nasty.

Non-saturated essential fatty acids omega-3, 6 and 9 are just about the very best things you can consume in order to grow great hair. Just like vitamin C, these fats are called 'essential' fatty acids because we cannot produce them ourselves and so we must rely on sourcing them from within our diets. They help to regulate hormones (including the hormones that if left unchecked can cause hair thinning and loss), increase good HDL cholesterol, improve circulation, boost cellular repair and reduce inflammation. All of these things not only benefit the body as a whole but really help your scalp and its follicles to produce top-quality hair. Cold-water fish such as salmon, trout, sardines and mackerel are all excellent – not to mention tasty – sources of healthy fats. Plus, they pack a protein punch too.

Unless you have been living under a rock for the last few years there is no way you would not have noticed the meteoric rise in popularity of coconut oil. There are literally hundreds of thousands of blog posts, YouTube videos and articles claiming coconut as a cure-all for a myriad of skin conditions, stubborn weight problems and – of course – hair issues.

Some of these stories are absolute nonsense and others are on to something. Coconut oil contains caprylic and lauric acids, which have been shown to support immunity (a well-functioning immune system is good news for new hair growth), while lauric acid is known to have antimicrobial properties, which are useful in the war against hair loss.

You can use coconut oil much in the same way as you would a pre-shampoo mask, by applying it all over your scalp and down to the tips of your hair and leaving it to work its magic for a few hours or even overnight, but you can also eat it. Thanks to its megastar status many recipes now incorporate coconut oil in place of other fats and you can even use it to cook with instead of regular oil.

COMPLEX CARBOHYDRATES

Low-carbohydrate and zero-carbohydrate diets dominated much of the nineties and hair really paid the price for it. The body breaks down complex carbohydrates and uses them for energy; without a good supply of them the body instead looks to stored proteins for its fuel. Restricting or eliminating complex carbohydrates for too long can result in hair loss. However, complex carbohydrates shouldn't be confused with simple, sugar-laden refined carbohydrates – like white bread and pasta, cakes and pastries – which don't contribute in any way to the condition of your hair – or indeed your health – and wreak havoc with your blood-sugar levels.

To get your fill of complex carbohydrates enjoy wholegrain bread and cereals, bulgar wheat, baked beans (check the sugar content), peas, parsnips, barley, oatmeal, legumes, fresh fruit, and brown rice and pasta. If you're eating a potato, eat the skin as well to make the most of the complex carbohydrates stored there too.

ZINC

Experts credit zinc with everything from supporting the division of hair-follicle cells and boosting healthier hair growth to strengthening the follicles' protein structures and preventing shedding and hair loss. Others suggest that it may even treat dandruff (it is for this reason that you'll often find zinc in anti-dandruff shampoos). Oysters, nuts, eggs, chickpeas, spinach and sweet potatoes are all sources of zinc.

BIOTIN

Biotin, a B vitamin, is another one of these 'essential' components that our bodies so desperately need but cannot produce. This clever B vitamin is a bit of a multitasker; it helps the body make use of carbohydrates, fats and amino acids and by doing this it supports healthy hair growth and minimises how much hair falls out before its time. So if you're deficient in biotin you may experience some hair loss, but that's not the worst of it: in some cases it can leach your hair of colour and make you go grey earlier than you should. Vitamin B is present in smallish amounts in egg yolks, liver, cauliflower, mushrooms, avocados, beans, nuts, salmon and pork.

SNACKING

As I mentioned, hair cells are the second-fastest-dividing cells in the human body and as such need a near-constant supply of energy. The energy stores that your hair follicles draw on for fuel are usually running on empty around four hours after your last meal. This is why snacking in between meals is absolutely essential if you want incredible hair. Unfortunately that should not be a chocolate-bar-shaped snack. Complex carbohydrates are your hair follicles' best source of fuel at these times so snack away on a handful of nuts, wholemeal crackers, some raw vegetables such as carrots with hummus (chickpeas are also a complex carbohydrate) or wholemeal bread.

WATER

I know I'm not telling you anything new here but suffice to say, drinking plenty of water is non-negotiable for great hair. Drinking a sufficient amount of water is necessary for every aspect of your health and it's no less important when it comes to the condition, look and feel of your hair. If you allow your body to become chronically dehydrated your scalp (just like the rest of your skin) will become dry, flaky, easily irritated, itchy and uncomfortable and you'll most likely develop dandruff. Water keeps your scalp moisturised, supple and calm while at the same time it also assists with cellular communication, which keeps your follicles efficient and in tip-top condition. Aim for 1.5 to 2 litres of water a day, more if you live in a hot and humid environment or work out a lot. There's no excuse for allowing yourself to become dehydrated.

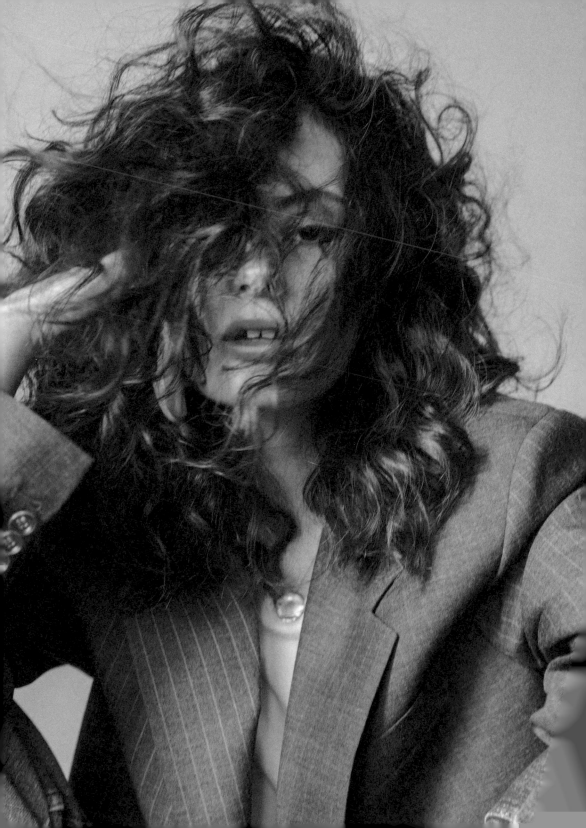

HAIR HEROES

Depending on the state of your existing diet, implementing the previous changes will either be a cinch or an absolute nightmare. I would hate for you to try and do everything at once only to cave in because it feels unachievable. If what I have talked about looks very different from what you eat at the moment, ease yourself in slowly and incorporate the following heroes into your diet to begin with. It's certainly a step in the right direction.

Sunflower seeds are just such an incredible source of goodness. These unassuming – but tasty – seeds contain vitamin E, omega-6, biotin, potassium, zinc, iron, B vitamins, magnesium and calcium. Sprinkle them over your salads and vegetables (they add a great crunch), mix them into oats and smoothies or just keep a bag of them in your desk drawer to snack on during the day.

Cold-water fish such as salmon, trout and sardines are packed with omega-3 fatty acids and protein.

Oats boast iron, fibre, omega-3 fatty acids and polyunsaturated fatty acids. They also release their energy slowly so believe the hype when they say they fill you up for the day.

Mighty greens like spinach, kale and broccoli offer up a double whammy of iron and vitamin C. Remember, they can lose much of their vitamin content when they're cooked so eat them as close to raw as you can stomach.

Nuts are good sources of vitamin E, protein, B vitamins, zinc, iron, magnesium, calcium and potassium. Mix them in with some sunflower seeds and you've got the ultimate hair-friendly snack.

SUPPLEMENTS

Without a doubt it is far better to get our vitamins and minerals from our diet. That said, there are some that can benefit from being supplemented too. Supplements should never replace a healthy, balanced diet but they can enhance one. The below are supplements that trichologists and dermatologists usually recommend for boosting the health of your hair. If you have *any* concerns speak to your health practitioner or a qualified dietician first.

Omega-3 fatty acids: We know that these are vital for a healthy, balanced scalp and glossy, beautiful hair. Look for omega-3s that have come from a marine source and have an EPA/DHA amount between 200 and 700 milligrams per capsule. The higher the dosage the greater the concentration of hair-loving omega-3.

Biotin: This is a vitamin that is most definitely worth supplementing as the foods in which it can be found tend to contain only small amounts of it. Try a daily supplement containing 500g of biotin.

Vitamin D: As I mentioned, experts agree that the majority of the world's population is deficient in vitamin D to some extent. If you live in the Northern Hemisphere then it is likely that you will go months on end without any concentrated sun exposure and so your need will be greater than, say, someone living in the tropics. Likewise, the paler your skin the easier your body finds it to create vitamin D when it comes into contact with the sun's rays. But if your skin is dark it is unlikely to absorb sufficient UV rays to create a large quantity of vitamin D so again, your need is great.

According to experts, the typical government-recommended daily allowance in most countries falls woefully short of the amount we *should* be taking and so they suggest a very minimum of 1,000 International Units (IU) a day for a healthy adult.

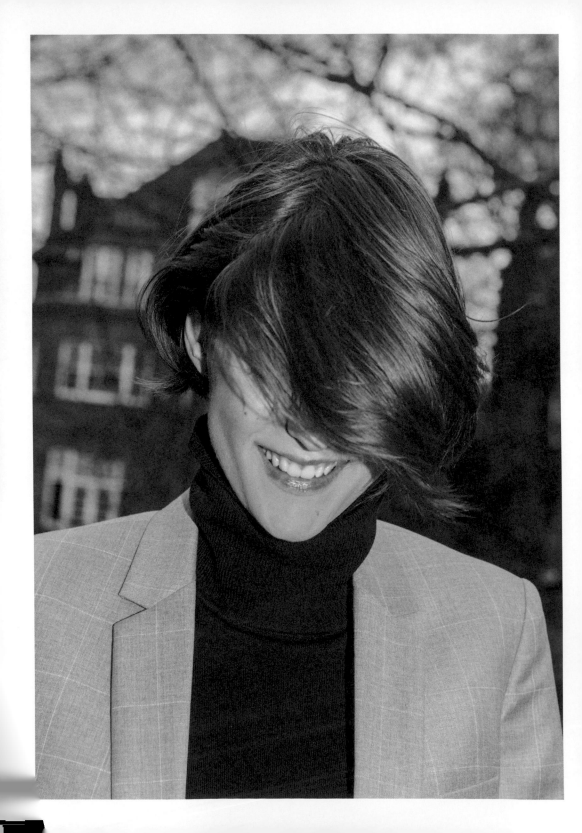

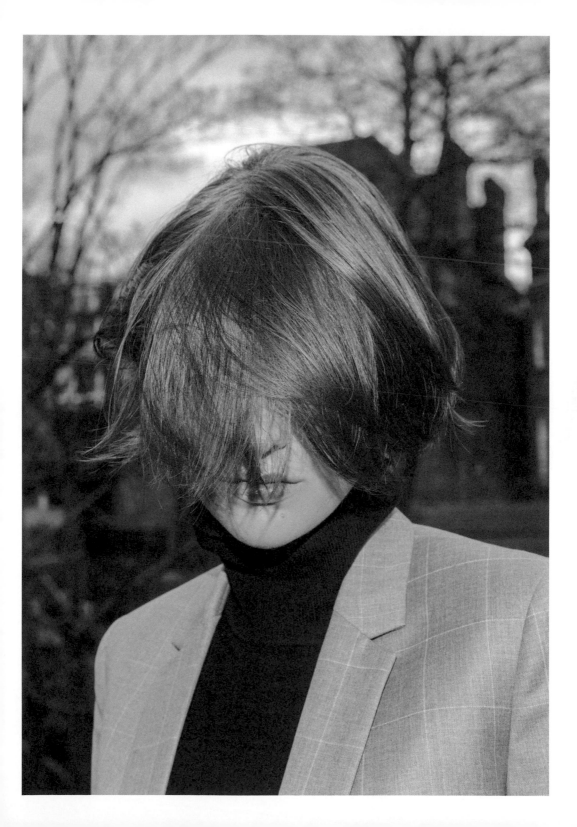

EXERCISE

Moderate cardio boosts blood circulation, which is good for your scalp and of course it boosts your general health; if your body is in good working order it has no excuse not to channel nutrients to your scalp and hair follicles. It's a very different story, however, for chronic over-exercisers. Excessive exercise over a long period has been shown to subject the body to stress, which in turns leads to inflammation, which is damaging to hair and the scalp.

Swimming in chlorinated pools is terribly damaging to hair. The chemicals – whilst necessary to keep the water clean – can dry out and irritate your scalp and weaken and dehydrate your hair. Try rinsing your hair with non-chlorinated water before entering the pool. The plain water will absorb into the hair shaft and fill it up so that it takes on less of the chlorinated water. Alternatively, wear a swimming cap to properly shield your hair. But in both cases be sure to use an intensive mask with proteins and conditioners such as shea butter afterwards to re-strengthen.

STRESS

Stress can have a profound effect on the health and appearance of hair. Juggling a career with a family and social life can take its toll on even the most together person. All it takes is a sudden difficult spell at work, or a romantic relationship to break down out of the blue, to send your stress levels through the roof. Chronic stress can result in hormonal changes that force follicles out of their growth phase and into a resting and shedding phase. This ultimately means that there will be less hair on your head. But the results of stress are not immediately obvious and will show up around six to twelve weeks afterwards.

Of course, in times of extreme stress, we also often neglect to take good care of ourselves – it's human nature. Sleep becomes elusive and a healthy, balanced diet goes out of the window. Stress can also cripple your digestive system so even if you are eating wonderfully hair-friendly foods, your body can't take what it needs from them.

When some people are under stress they can resort to trichotillomania as a coping mechanism. This sees the sufferer give in to an overwhelming urge to pluck out their own hair. Some experts even suggest that chronic stress is a contributing factor in alopecia areata, in which the body's own immune system attacks healthy follicles and causes hair to fall out.

For many of us, stress isn't something easily avoided but there are steps that can be taken to minimise the fallout (so to speak). Mindfulness is growing in popularity, as is Green Therapy, which essentially involves spending as much time in nature as possible, while low-intensity exercise like yoga has been shown to effectively ease stress in some. Feeling stressed is certainly nothing to be ashamed of and if you are struggling to cope with it, or you are experiencing something like trichotillomania or alopecia areata, then you absolutely should speak to a medical professional for support and guidance.

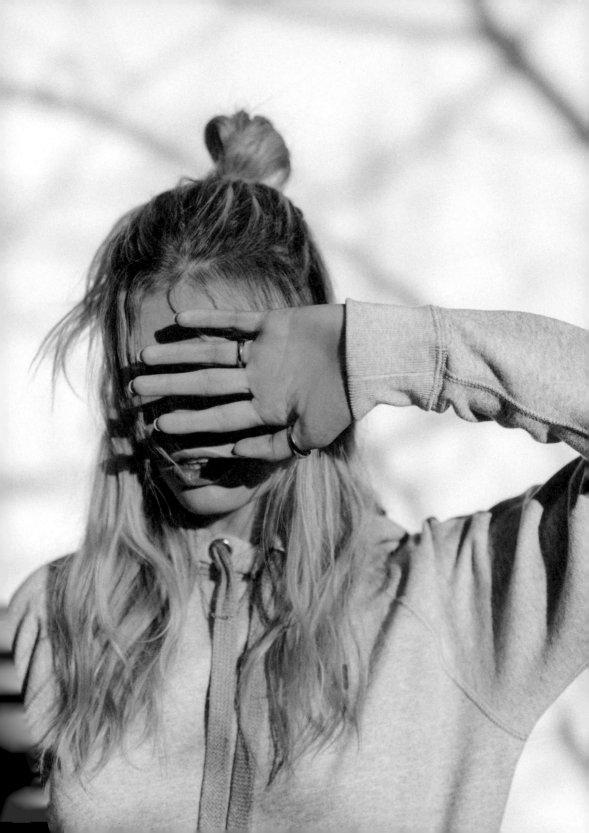

HAIR
WOES

'Why not try embracing them rather than hiding them?'

We *all* have things we don't like about our hair – women are certainly not alone in this. Whether it's a stubborn cowlick that scuppers your best efforts at a blow dry, perpetual frizz, a thinning hairline or a greasy fringe, there is always an element or two that bothers us to the point of being irrational – while other people probably don't even notice it. Let's see what we can do about this, shall we? Here are your most common issues and what you can do about them.

I HAVE A COWLICK

I know that having a cowlick – or a 'hair whorl' as some people call them – can be incredibly infuriating when you're styling your hair. Thankfully, they're easier to tame than you might think and it doesn't require a fancy brush or a pair of hair straighteners. When you're in that crucial rough-drying phase, grasp the cowlick in between your fingers as if your hand was a comb. Direct the airflow from your hairdryer directly at the offending section of hair, aiming it in the direction you want the hair to fall. As you dry, gently pull and drag on the hair with your fingers so that there is constant tension on it.

I HAVE A DOUBLE CROWN

People assume that if you have a double crown then you have some kind of obstacle to cross when it comes to styling and cutting. But really it doesn't matter if you have a double crown or not and, despite what some hairstylists will tell you, a double crown makes no difference to how to style your hair and it doesn't influence what kind of cut you can have. Trust me – I have one.

MY HAIR IS ALWAYS FRIZZY

There are a few things you can do here to soften your frizz. First of all, make sure to apply a smoothing product like Hershesons Almost Everything Cream or John Frieda Frizz Ease to your hair while it is still wet. Then as you're drying it in, repeat the rough-drying process I mentioned before: use your hands as you would a giant comb and capture, drag and pull your hair as it dries, with the direction of the airflow from your hairdryer facing downwards – this will encourage the cuticle layer to lie flat and smooth. As you're drying your hair you may notice a little steam. I know this usually sends alarm bells and it's easy to think that you're burning your hair but, trust me, you are not. What is happening is some of the oils in the products are evaporating off and this is essential to create that silky finish to the hair.

Never brush your hair when it's dry; this will only make your hair frizzier and more static. I often see women and fellow hairdressers laboriously blow-dry hair until it is silky and smooth, only to run the brush through it again once it is dry and set off more static. It's infuriating. Only brush your hair while you're drying it, and as soon as your hair is dry put the brush down.

Alternatively, a Permanent Blow Dry – which uses keratin to restructure hair and reduce frizz – could be really useful for you. You can get all your hair done or if you find you only frizz up in certain areas – such as around your hairline – then just have the permanent treatment applied there.

MY HAIR IS BREAKING

Breakage is usually a result of overdoing chemical treatments. If you have had bleach applied on top of bleach, and you straighten or tong your hair every day, then it is not too much of a surprise that it's starting to snap. Scale right back on your chemical treatments and always, *always* use a heat-defence spray on your hair before applying heat to it – better yet, reread Your Hair Routine and take note of where I talk about air-drying your hair; cutting back on the number of days in the week that you use heat styling can only be a good thing.

Breakage can also be down to deficiencies within your diet so I suggest rereading Great Hair from the Inside Out.

Sadly, if your hair is already breaking there's not a whole lot you can do except limit the damage. A good cut should remove a lot of the broken ends and prevent splits from travelling up the hair shaft while a regimen of restorative protein masks – such as a weekly dose of Philip Kingsley Elasticizer – will restore *some* of the strength your hair has lost.

I HAVE A PPD ALLERGY

PPD (or technically, para-phenylenediamine) is a chemical found in permanent hair dyes. Some people can have a very serious allergic reaction to PPD showing up as stinging, blistering, swelling and a rash. On occasion a PPD allergy can result in anaphylaxis, which can prove fatal. What makes PPD particularly challenging is that some women may develop an allergy to it out of the blue. Your colourist must do a patch test forty-eight hours before your first colour to ensure you're not showing any signs of a reaction.

Vegetable dyes and henna are good natural alternatives to regular hair colour though they don't provide the same kind of coverage or depth of colour as a chemical version.

If you want to switch up your hair colour by just a shade or two, I suggest you think about having some hair fillers (minute hair extensions) in a slightly different colour from your own put in a few places; this will add depth or lift to your natural colour without having to add any colourant to your own hair. Granted, fillers will not cover grey but they are an excellent option for adding some tonal variation.

I GET DANDRUFF

You're not alone, dandruff is a surprisingly common skin condition. Contrary to what some people believe, dandruff is not down to poor hygiene – though it can look worse if you don't wash your hair regularly. There are a number of reasons why you might have dandruff – it could be related to eczema, psoriasis or dermatitis – and not only does it look unpleasant but it can also leave your scalp feeling tight and itchy too. Zinc pyrithione (ZPT) is a very good anti-dandruff treatment as it treats the underlying cause of dandruff as well as eliminating flakes and soothing irritation. You'll find it in anti-dandruff

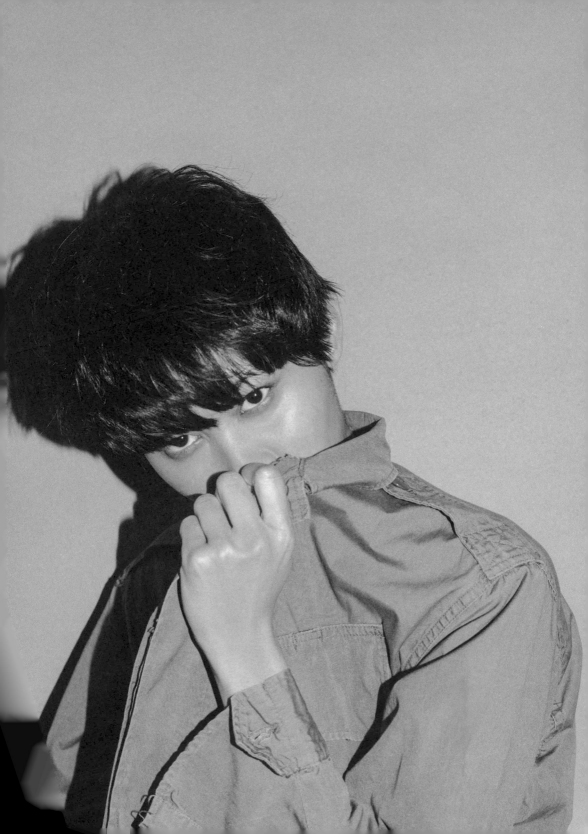

shampoos including – an oldie but a goodie – Head & Shoulders. If after a month your skin is still shedding and the itching is not getting better it's time to see your GP or health practitioner.

MY HAIR IS SO FLAT

Naturally thin and fine hair can lie close to your scalp and look unflatteringly limp. At the risk of sounding like a broken record, you really can't underestimate the importance of a great cut if you have fine, lifeless hair. A great cut will create volume seemingly out of nowhere. The best time to maximise this is when you're rough-drying your hair after washing it. If you're up to it, try using a round-barrelled brush as you dry to lift your hair away from your roots to create height. Aim the nozzle of your hairdryer directly at the roots to create as much volume as possible.

If using a round brush is likely to lead to a mass of knots then your hands can do just as good a job. As you're rough-drying use your hand like an oversized comb to grab and lift your hair away from your roots. Keep alternating the direction to really maximise lift at the roots. A mist of Elnett at the end will help to hold the shape for as long as possible.

For a more long-term solution, look into a perm. At Hershesons we do a perm that is just designed to add thickness and volume. Instead of setting the hair around rollers and creating a curl, we lightly plait the hair so that it creates bulk. Not all hairdressers offer this kind of perm so you would need to ask, or alternatively visit London for an appointment with us.

MY HAIR IS MIXTURE OF TEXTURES

It's more common than you think to have a couple of different textures happening in your hair. My advice is to decide which part you love the most and enhance that. For example, if you have wavy hair underneath and straighter hair on top, just lightly tong a few sections around the surface of your hair to marry the two textures together. Often it's the sections of hair around the hairline that wildly differ in texture. If this is the case, a Permanent Blow Dry applied just to those sections should do the trick. The worst thing you can do is try and change every hair on your head.

MY FRINGE DOESN'T DRY
THE WAY I WANT IT TO

Most people tend to over-work and over-dry their fringe, which is a recipe for disaster. They wrap it around a large-barrelled brush and they pull it as it dries and what happens? It pings right out and looks a complete mess. The secret to a perfectly styled fringe is to treat it gently. Put your round brush underneath the hair and allow the fringe just to rest on top. As you dry your hair, roll the brush beneath without dragging. The finish will be far softer and prettier.

MY FRINGE GETS GREASY
IN THE AFTERNOON

It's to be expected that a fringe becomes a little limp as the day wears on as the oils produced on your skin transfer from your forehead to your hair. Never leave the house without a travel-sized can of dry shampoo – it's the best and quickest way to absorb a little bit of that oil and refresh your fringe on the go. Keep the can a good distance from your hair so it doesn't clump and spray your fringe from underneath, and buff the product through with your fingers.

MY HAIR STARTS SMOOTH BUT
PUFFS UP BY LUNCHTIME

I suggest investing in a Permanent Blow Dry, which uses keratin to rework the structure of your hair without changing its texture and shape too much. What it *will* do, however, is make your hair more resistant to humidity so it's less likely to puff up. A mini can of Elnett is always a good thing to carry in your bag to tame your hair mid-afternoon too.

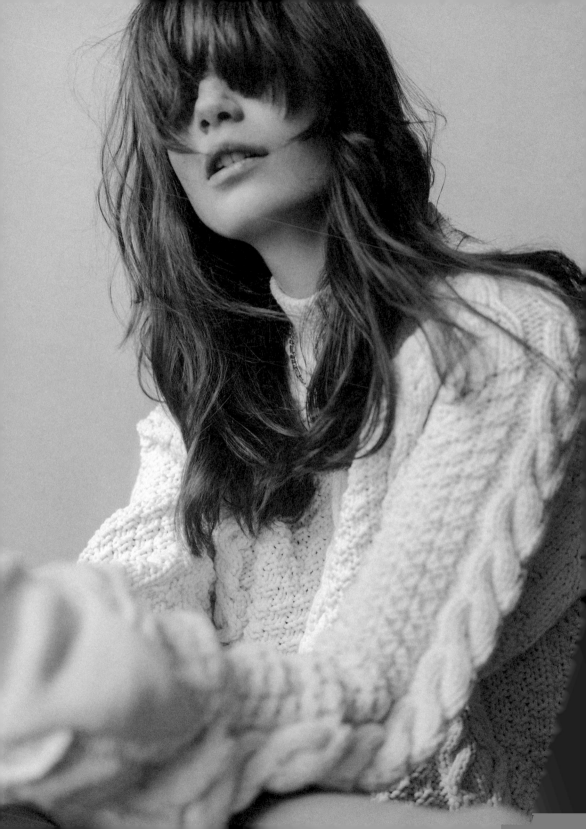

WHAT SHOULD I DO WITH MY SPLIT ENDS?

I don't suggest trimming them yourself; you may have a light hand with your scissors but there's a chance that you will concentrate your efforts in one place and imbalance your cut. If you don't want to remove any length ask your hairdresser for an invisible trim. They will twist sections of your hair to make the splits stand out on end and then *carefully* run their scissors parallel down the length of the hair to just to snip off the splits.

MY FINE HAIR IS GREASY

Dry shampoo is the obvious answer for a quick and instant fix but it won't get to the cause of the problem. Take a look at your shampoo and conditioner: are you using the right ones? (See What You Need, What You Don't.) There's a chance that you're using products containing heavy oils and butters that your fine hair can't cope with. When your hair feels greasy it's tempting to wash it every day, but this can stress your scalp, strip it of its natural oils and provoke it into producing even more sebum in response. The result is a vicious cycle of grease. If you're currently washing your hair every day, scale it back to every other day and see if that makes a difference.

MY HAIR GETS STATIC IN THE OFFICE

Office air conditioning can be very drying, which is a nightmare situation for static hair. Do not brush your hair when it is dry, as it will make it even more static and prone to frizz – instead just lightly mist it with Elnett. Elnett is a great product to layer up during the day as needed because it remains soft.

MY CURLS LACK DEFINITION

There's a really simple, if a little traditional, fail-safe technique to bring definition to natural and permed curls alike and that's a diffuser. Apply some Hershesons Almost Everything Cream to your hair while it is still wet and then drop your hair in sections into an upturned diffuser attachment on your hairdryer. Don't be tempted to touch your hair too much – you might disrupt your curl pattern – just leave it pooled in the diffuser until it dries. Then simply separate out your curls with your hands.

WHAT SHOULD I DO WITH MY FLYAWAYS?

I love baby hairs. Why not try embracing them rather than hiding them? Push them a little further onto your forehead and rub them in between your thumb and forefinger to bring some shape and control to them. The alternative is to flatten them with some hairspray and a dry toothbrush or a hairdresser's neck brush, which is fatter and denser, but I think it's far more fun to play them up.

WHAT CAN I DO ABOUT GREYS THAT CROP UP IN BETWEEN APPOINTMENTS?

Don't pluck them out. I'm not saying that because two will grow in its place (which, FYI, is just an old wives' tale); it's just an unnecessary and counterintuitive thing to do considering that most women lose some hair density as they get older. Also, here's the thing: while they may be the first thing you see when you look in the mirror I guarantee no one else really notices them.

Shampoos and conditioners that refresh bottled colour are good for in between appointments. Try John Frieda's range of shampoos and conditioners like Brilliant Brunette and Radiant Red. For an instant solution try Color Wow Root Cover Up, a pigmented powder that you pat onto your roots with a brush. It's very subtle and cleverly hides the odd grey hair.

SHOULD I EVER TRIM MY OWN FRINGE?

No. That's what your hairdresser is for.

MY HAIR EXTENSIONS MATT AT THE ROOTS

Next time ask your stylist for Remi hair extensions; they're slightly more expensive than other extensions but the hair has been collected in a way that allows it all to run in the same direction and they are so much less likely to matt.

Also, make sure you brush your hair every day when you're wearing extensions. To not do so will encourage the hair to knot and clump in places. This is the only time you should ever brush your hair while it is dry.

MY HAIR CAN'T HOLD CURLS OR WAVES

Some virgin hair or freshly washed hair is resistant to curling and when it *does* curl it's quick to fall out. Try not to wave your hair on the same day as you wash it – the curl will take much better if your hair is a day or two past its last wash. Alternatively, make sure you use a curling tong that has a clamp; this allows you to trap the hair directly against the barrel so it's more likely to bend. Getting the right cut can greatly improve your curling success rate; a few hidden layers here and there will make it much easier to tong.

HOW CAN I HIDE MY THINNING HAIRLINE?

A thinning hairline in women is not uncommon, especially if you are someone who likes to wear your hair up a lot as the tension can result in it becoming sparse. Adding a few hair fillers (extensions) around your hairline can bulk up your hair but if you want a more temporary solution buy yourself some Color Wow Root Cover Up. Use the brush to pat the powder over the thin areas in your hairline and it will give the illusion of more hair. There are eight shades to choose from so you should get a good colour match.

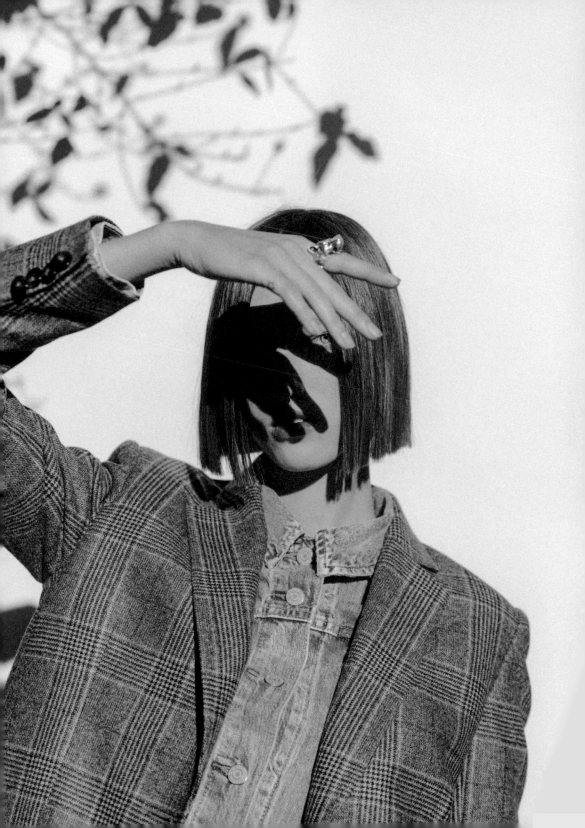

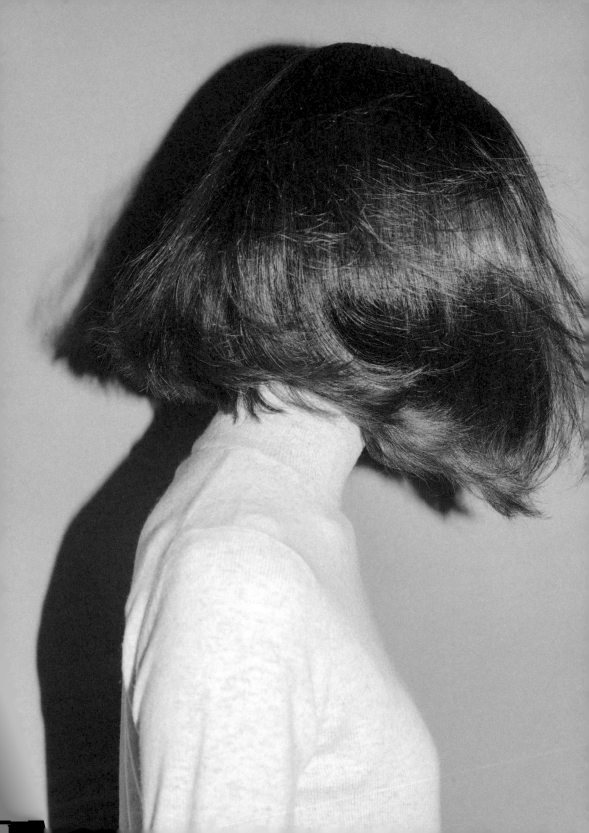

THE
HERSHESONS

'Back then this was the first, and it was groundbreaking'

Hair is in the Hersheson DNA. I grew up in my dad's salons and from as early as the age of four I knew I wanted to be just like him. Daniel is the founder of our brand but his own father, Jack, was a hairdresser too, so hair is in his blood, just like mine. Daniel often says that as a hairdresser his job has always been to make people look great regardless of their age, their hair type or their personality, and that is what Hershesons still stands for today.

My dad left school at fifteen to train at the Xavier Wenger salon in Knightsbridge. By the time he was just twenty-one he already had his own salon called Neville Daniel in Marylebone with a couple of partners. It was here that he met my mum Ruth when she came in for an appointment.

I remember, later on, watching my dad in his salon and thinking that he was not a typical hairdresser. Back then hair salons had a weird vibe; hairdressers did the same haircuts year in, year out, and they just never moved their style on. But with my dad, his work was so much more modern than that. He was constantly changing and I wondered how he knew *what* to change – how did he know where things were going next?

In around 1991–92 he came up with this shaggy, rock 'n' roll bob – which later on became quite a trend – and he was literally the only person doing it at the time. This was when supermodels were still kind of influential but the taste in London was definitely moving towards grunge. The style got picked up and other hairdressers started doing their own version until inevitably it became something very different and almost a little vulgar. But he brought to life this amazing style out of nowhere and somehow instinctively knew that it was the right thing at the right time. I remember thinking it was such a shame that salons in general had this awful cheesy reputation when he was doing some really cool work.

By 1992 my dad and his partners had gone their separate ways and he was opening the first Daniel Hersheson salon on Conduit Street in London. I was there all the time, sweeping, washing hair, tidying up and practising on blocks – which look like weird dolls' heads – in the old barber section that used to be on the first floor.

I would spend ages looking at the work of legendary hairstylists Sam McKnight, Eugene Souleiman and Guido Palau, at this world of fashion that seemed very closed off and untouchable. But the styles they created were so cool and about as far as possible as you could get from what people associated with salon hairdressing. I asked myself why these two worlds couldn't coexist. Why couldn't you have the coolness and relevance and modernity of the hairstyles being created at the shows and in magazines, but in the salon? I couldn't understand why the two things had to be mutually exclusive. I was actually quite ashamed that salons had this really dodgy and cheesy reputation. They just weren't relevant.

I became a full-time stylist when I was nineteen and once qualified I knew that the first step to changing this old-fashioned perception of salons was to establish myself as a session stylist and work in both fashion and the salon. That way I could bring some of coolness from that world into what we were doing for our clients.

I begged for work experience behind the camera until a client of mine – who as fortune had it happened to be a photographer's agent – gave me my first break at the age of twenty-one working on a campaign for Missoni. The rest, as they say, is history and I have gone on to work for French, Italian, American and British *Vogue*, *W*, the *Gentlewoman*, *Self Service*, *i-D* and *Love* and with photographers like Mert Alas and Marcus Piggott, David Sims, Alasdair McLellan, Collier Schorr, Walter Pfeiffer, Jamie Hawkesworth and Paolo Roversi. I have had the privilege to work on some incredible campaigns for Missoni, Bottega Veneta, Armani and Giuseppe Zanotti, and with a raft of well-known faces including Keira Knightley, Sienna Miller, Emma Watson and Rachel Weisz and, of course, Victoria Beckham, who generously offered to write the foreword for this book.

I truly feel that at Hershesons we have had a lot to do with bringing together these two worlds that were for the longest time poles apart, and the people who have been with us along the way and have since gone on to establish their own businesses and brands – like Alex Brownsell, George Northwood, Rudi Lewis, Lyndell Mansfield, Syd Hayes, Tina Outen and Larry King – have really helped to bridge that gap even further.

At Hershesons we quickly started making waves. Other hairdressers were doing a lot of daytime TV and hair shows, so we decided early on that we wouldn't be involved in either of those things. It would have brought us recognition and we knew that doing it our way was going to be much harder, but we also knew that it would give us more integrity. It ended up being more about what we said no to than what we said yes to that earned us our reputation.

Around 1997–98 my name started getting out there as a session stylist so we thought, let's do our own photos for in-salon but make them look like fashion pictures. The imagery typically used in-salon then was so out-dated and boring; we decided we wanted to shoot ours full length and make sure the hair was moving and looked touchable. I wasn't particularly experienced at that point but I had a clear idea of where I wanted to take things. What really started to set us apart from everyone else was when we decided to give our cuts their own names – something so simple that everybody does now, but at the time was virtually unheard of. Our first one was called 'The Shunk', which I think was meant to be a shaggy monk-like look. It was a take on a shag but a bit more rounded and very, very ironed.

Straight hair had become something that everyone wanted; it was on the catwalk and in magazines so we brought it into the salon and became the first people to introduce the straightening iron to the UK. This was huge news at the time and I remember the *Telegraph* dedicating an entire page to this new look we had created.

Trying to get your cuts and looks out there for people to see before the internet and social media was quite tricky if you were not doing TV appearances, and we decided we wanted to work with models so our looks could be seen in shoots and on the catwalk. Storm modelling agency started sending us their new faces for cuts and it was a win-win situation for everyone. For the models it meant getting a decent cut and colour for their portfolio; for us it reinforced our connection to the fashion industry if our clients could see models having their hair done in-salon.

We were the first salon to work with a model agency this way and it really paid off. For some models (think along the lines of Edie Campbell and Agyness Deyn) all it takes is one defining cut to elevate their career to new heights, leading to more shows, more magazine covers and more campaigns. Soon we had models like Lily Cole, Alexa Chung and Rosie

Huntington-Whiteley in the salon and this led to a yearly collaboration with Storm sponsored by L'Oréal Professionnel, in which we would take twenty of their models and create pictures that we could use in the salon and they could use in their portfolios.

Things really started to take off. In 2004 we opened our second flagship salon in London, on the fourth floor of Harvey Nichols in Knightsbridge, and in January of 2006 we had another first; we launched a Hershesons Blow Dry Bar in Topshop's flagship store on Oxford Circus. Blow dry bars are ten a penny now but back then this was the first, and it was groundbreaking. For £19 and in just thirty minutes, women could pick a look from the menu and have it brought to life there and then, in-store, or for £15 and in just fifteen minutes, they could have their hair refreshed and blow-dried without even getting it wet. Since then we have gone on to open blow dry bars in some of the most prestigious locations and department stores in the UK including Selfridges in London and Birmingham, and Harvey Nichols in Knightsbridge.

The years have gone by in a blur of launches, innovations in-salon, celebrity clients, red carpets and magazine shoots and now, with the launch of Almost Everything Cream in 2018 (our first ever wet styling product that has been in development for years), we're really starting to get to the bottom of what our clients – and women in general – need for their hair. We're hoping that by eliminating many of the products gathering dust in bathrooms everywhere we can make a real difference to how women approach their styling and cut back on the time it takes to get ready to boot.

In 2018 we said goodbye to the Daniel Hersheson salon on Conduit Street. It had been at the heart of the brand for twenty-six years but change is exciting and we were ready for something fresh. Now Hershesons can be found on Berners Street in Fitzrovia, one of the most buzzing and exciting places in London.

Ultimately, what our brand has come to be known for, I hope, is our ability to make women look and feel great. We would hate for our clients to feel intimidated or bamboozled by hairdressing jargon, or for our stylists to be cutting hair in some formulaic way when, in fact, really a lot of feeling goes into a cut and knowing when something looks great or when something

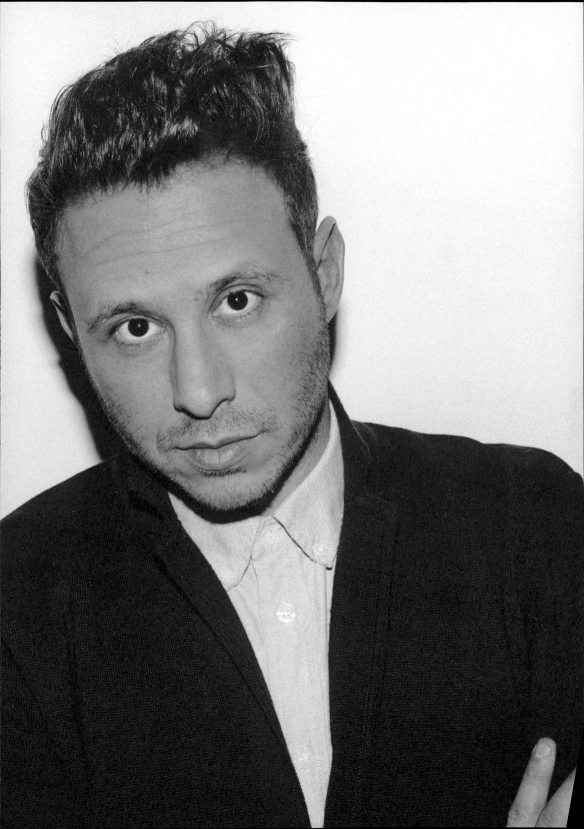

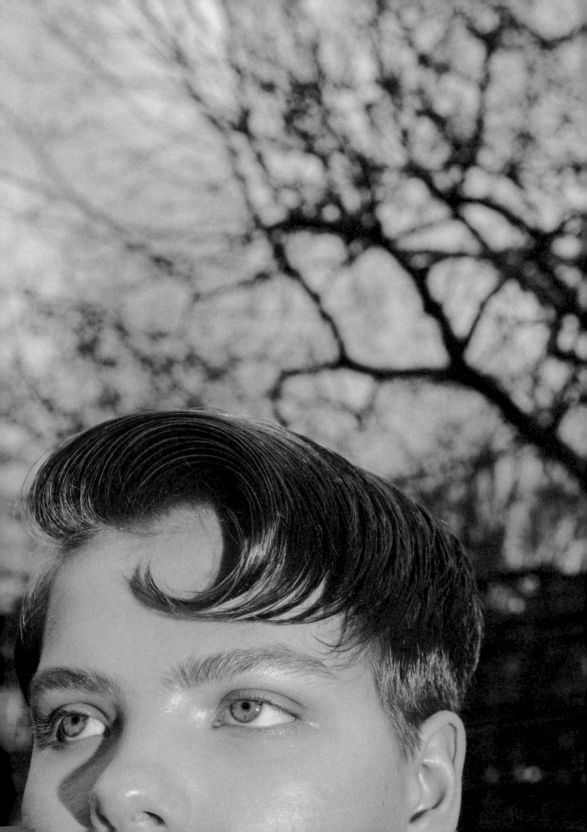

doesn't. There is no formula to a great cut or great hair. This is where *Great Hair Days* comes in; this book should make your life easier and strip away some of the mystery around hair.

Some aspects of hairdressing are still stuck in the Dark Ages when it comes to training. Hairdressers are taught to be 'technically' perfect, to be able to execute a precise cut set within tight parameters. That's not how we work and it's not how we teach our trainees. I always says to our assistants that I really couldn't care less if they're 'technically' not that brilliant; knowing how you want someone to look is far more important. As stylists, we have to be able to visualise what we're going to create before we even pick up a pair of scissors. I remember renowned hairstylist Guido Palau telling me once, 'I always think about what it should look like and only then do I worry about how I'm going to do it.' That is how we think here at Hershesons. So many hairdressers get off on the technique rather than the end result.

My dad likens the process to designing a dress. 'You start with the picture in your head – you know from the get-go what it is that you're going to create, what it's going to look like. Then you work out how you're going to make the bloody thing.' You would be surprised just how many hairdressers don't even start with that image in their mind; they kind of make it up as they go along, which reflects badly not just on them but also on the whole salon and everyone else working there. Nothing makes me prouder than when I see great work going out the door, and on the reverse, nothing makes me feel more shit than when the work is bad.

I'm blessed. I love every single day of my job, even the stressful ones. Whether I am cutting hair, developing products, or working on-set or backstage, I still find what I do a thrill. To my regret I don't get to cut hair in the salon very often any more but I try to make an appearance on the shop floor at least once a week. Above all I still love cutting hair and, like my dad, I do not believe in boundaries or rules. You don't have to be a certain age or look a certain way to carry off a hairstyle. Everyone can have great hair, every day.

Luke Hersheson, 2018

TIMELINE

1992

Dad opens our first flagship 'Daniel Hersheson' salon
in London on Conduit Street.

1997

I 'officially' join the company.

1998

After noticing a trend for poker-straight hair in New York and
on the catwalk, we introduce the first straightening iron to
the UK.

2002

We launch one of our all-time most successful styles,
'Wavy Gravy', consisting of loose and relaxed cool waves.
It's still on the menu today.

2003

We start to expand our range of tools and launch our first
hairdryer in Selfridges as part of a capsule collection.

2004

Our second London 'Daniel Hersheson' flagship salon
opens on the fourth floor of the iconic Knightsbridge
department store, Harvey Nichols.

2006

We break the mould and launch the world's first
blow dry bar in Topshop on Oxford Circus.

2010

We open the world's first hair apothecary, selling fun and
practical hairpieces and accessories.

2010

Our online store goes live.

2011

I scoop the award for Hair Icon at the Creative HEAD
Most Wanted awards.

2012

We launch the Hershesons Batiste dry shampoo and the Blow
Dry bus exclusive at *Vogue*'s Fashion Night Out in London.

2012

Our fourth blow dry bar opens in Selfridges, London.

2013

Our flagship Conduit Street salon undergoes a facelift.

2015

Another first: we launch the braid bar.

2018

We say farewell to 'Daniel Hersheson' on Conduit Street and
hello to the shiny and new 'Hershesons' on Berners Street.

2018

Finally, after twenty-five years, we launch our long-awaited and
eagerly anticipated wet styling product called
Almost Everything Cream.

2018

Our first book, *Great Hair Days & How to Have Them*,
is launched globally.

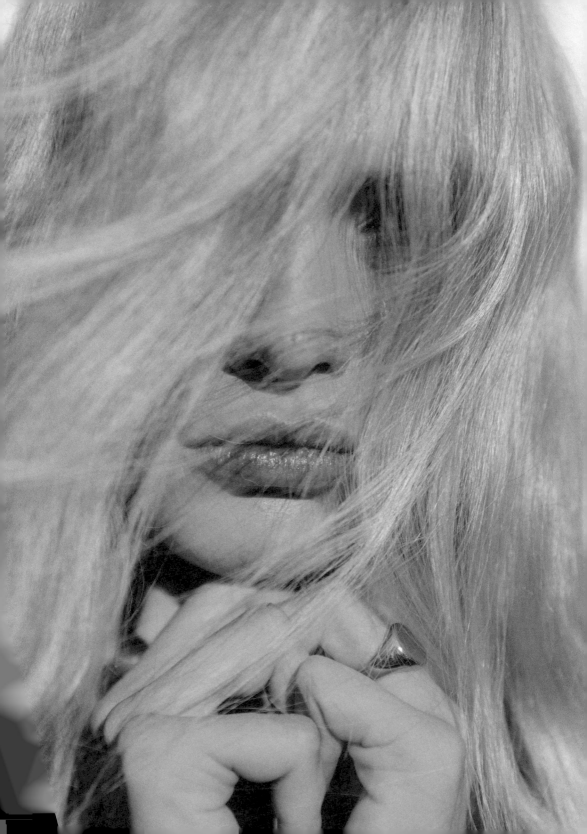

WHERE
TO
FIND
THE
COOLEST
HAIR

'Inspiration
can strike
anywhere'

As a hairdresser and someone who has to constantly come up with new ideas for shoots and celebrities, I am conditioned to look for inspiration everywhere I go. It's a necessary part of the job. I want you too to be surrounded by inspiration and to think creatively with your own style. This is where I find the coolest hair.

INSTAGRAM

I'm sure I'm not the only one who can begin scrolling through my Instagram feed only to notice forty-five minutes have flown by in the blink of an eye. Instagram feeds our voyeuristic tendencies and can be a brilliant source of inspiration. If you're a hairdresser or a colourist you're missing a trick if you're not on Instagram; it should be an extension of your portfolio and it's your best method of communication with people who are interested in what you do. If you love hair as much as I do, here's who you should follow.

@SamMcKnight1
Sam McKnight's Instagram serves up plenty of backstage insights from the likes of Chanel, Philosophy and Dries Van Noten, and throwback pictures from his archive sharing rare glimpses of his work with the Supers including Cindy Crawford and, of course, images of himself with Princess Diana when he was her hairstylist. But it's not all hair, in fact there's plenty for green thumbs too as he loves to share pictures of his envy-inducing garden.

@ClaireThomsonJonville
Claire is the ex-editor-in-chief of a French magazine called *Self Service*. Despite living in Paris, Claire is Scottish and I follow her because she just has the most fantastic taste. Her feed is like a thoughtfully refined edit of the most cool and inspirational images in fashion, cinema and music, plus a few travel shots thrown in for good measure. A typical line-up would be a

grainy picture of Sigourney Weaver in *Working Girl*, next to a moody black-and-white image of Monica Bellucci and a shot of Claudia Schiffer dressed head to toe in animal print at the height of the nineties. You just can't help but feel inspired.

@NicolaClarkeColour
Nicola is one of the hair-colouring greats and is renowned for her blondes. She tends to the tresses of everyone from Kate Winslet and Cate Blanchett to Emma Stone and Carey Mulligan so her feed runs like a who's who of Hollywood's leading ladies.

@hairbychristiaan
This is the account for legendary Dutch hairstylist Christiaan Houtenbos. His feed is wildly eclectic and you're just as likely to see a selfie as you are a picture of hair. He definitely keeps things interesting.

@alexsteinherr
Alessandra is a beauty influencer and associate creative and ex-beauty director at British *Glamour* magazine. I have been cutting Alex's hair for a very long time and she is always eager to embrace a new length or a change. Her feed is full of all things beauty and she shares insights into her own hair journey.

@SuiteCarolineSalon
This is the feed for a salon in New York's Soho neighbourhood that was started by colourist Lena Ott. Lena is an authority on colour and has had a long career working with models like Doutzen Kroes, dyeing wigs for music videos including Lady Gaga's 'Alejandro' and consulting for Alexander Wang. The feed is full of just really brilliant, really inspiring hair.

@TraceyCunningham1
Tracey owns Mèche Salon in Los Angeles and is the colourist to practically the whole of Hollywood. I'm not kidding. She colours Margot Robbie, practically the entire Kardashian/Jenner clan, Drew Barrymore and Gwyneth Paltrow. Rather than stylised editorial shots, Tracey's feed is actually quite candid and gives you an unfiltered insight into her work.

@cimmahony
Cim is a Danish hairdresser and I really like his feed. He has exceptional taste and his imagery is inspiring.

@garrennewyork
Hairstylist Garren is somewhat of a legend in the hair industry and that really shows in the images and videos he chooses to share on Instagram. His feed is just as likely to throw up a modern and bold cut as it is a flashback to George Michael's 'Freedom' music video for which he bleached and cut Linda Evangelista's hair.

@JuliaHobbs_
Julia Hobbs is the fashion news editor at British *Vogue*, a regular in Hershesons and, in my humble opinion, a modern hair muse. She is constantly changing her style but whatever her hair looks like it is always modern, fun and daring and speaks volumes about her personal style.

THE HERSHESONS ALUMNI

George of @GeorgeNorthwood and Alex Brownsell of @bleachlondon both came up through the Hershesons ranks and have gone on to launch their own exciting business ventures. George is worth a follow just to see the occasional snap of his dog Rex but there's also lots of behind-the-scenes stuff with the likes of Alexa Chung, Rosie Huntington-Whiteley and Alicia Vikander. You'll know Alex from her phenomenal brand Bleach, which was kind of at the forefront of the whole pastel-hair movement. Bleach's feed is the ultimate inspiration for anyone who loves to experiment with colour.

THE CURRENT HERSHESONS TEAM

I highly recommend that you follow @thehairbros, Sean Paul Nother and Nick Latham. Their feed is young, cool and fresh and full of really great hair. Also follow other Hershesons stylists including @mrjordangarrett (Jordan shares plenty of snaps of his celebrity clients), @adrian.at.hershesons and @Premlee_at_Hershesons.

And I would be remiss if I didn't toot our own horn too. Should you drop by @Hershesons and @LukeHersheson you'll get a glimpse of everything we're inspired by and some of our latest work.

ON THE WEB

Unfortunately, hair is not catered to online or on YouTube in the same way as other aspects of beauty such as make-up, and even some of the big beauty websites are still behind in how they show and talk about great hair. YouTube is great if you want to see a hairstyle in practice but it lacks engaging and quality content. Sure, this is disappointing but it does mean that there are opportunities for anyone who is enthusiastic about hair to start their own thing. If you're launching your own hair-skewed platform then I suggest finding your niche and really thinking about what sets your content and style apart from everyone else's. Make your videos or stories inspirational and engaging and as a session stylist I can tell you that you should never underestimate the value of great lighting. If you're going to be filming or shooting your own work make sure the production value is really good. After all, this is your craft and you need to do it justice.

So, while I wouldn't say we're spoilt for choice with digital destinations for hair, the ones that are doing it well are doing it very well. Bookmark these:

maneaddicts.com
Mane Addicts is a brilliant online resource for video tutorials, inspirational images and insightful stories. It's always one of the first websites to report on trends and it consistently puts out good Fashion Week coverage. Whether you're a budding stylist or colourist, or you just love reinventing and playing with your own hair, there is something there for you.

pinterest.com
What did we do before Pinterest? It's the most easily accessible and user-friendly site for inspirational hair images by a long shot. Thinking of having a fringe cut in but you're not sure which style you're learning towards? Type the word 'fringe' into Pinterest and you will have literally thousands upon thousands of options instantly at your fingertips. You can compile mood

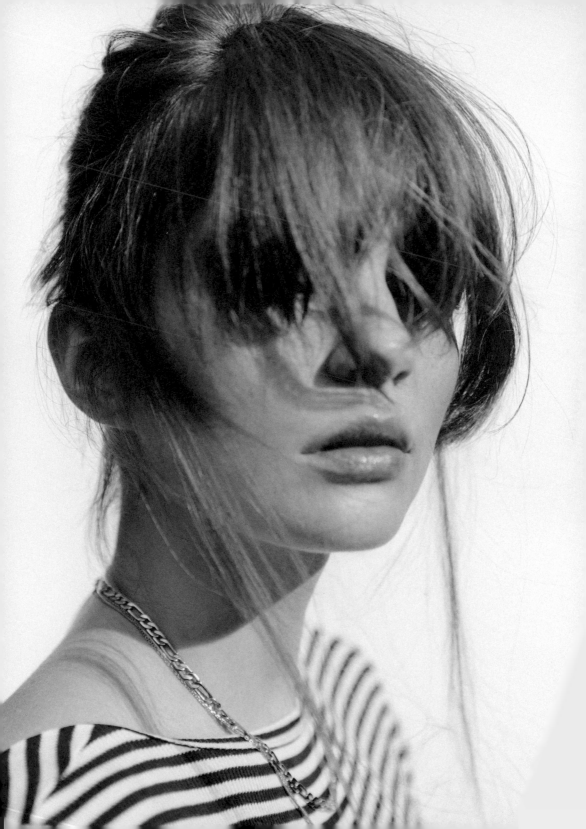

boards for every aspect of your hair from braids you love to colour you want to experiment with. You can download Pinterest onto your phone as an app too because inspiration can strike anywhere.

salihughesbeauty.com

If you want no-nonsense beauty advice then head over to Sali's site. Sali is a beauty columnist for the *Guardian* and she really cuts the crap. She has a huge following of loyal readers because they trust her to give it to them straight. If you want an honest opinion on a hair product, or you just want to read an excellent piece of beauty journalism, this website is definitely one to add to your favourites.

creativeheadmag.com

Creative Head is a brilliant resource for anyone in the hair industry. It's a place where you can lose yourself in trends, and videos that go on-set with various stylists, and all the latest news and goings-on. *Creative Head* is also a print magazine and if you're studying hair or training to become a stylist I definitely recommend you subscribe to it.

BOOKS AND MAGAZINES

Trawling Instagram and Pinterest is all well and good but sometimes the very best kind of inspiration is still to be found in a book. I have a rather sizeable collection containing the work of some acclaimed fashion photographers that I go back to time and time again when I need to feel inspired. Some photographers just know hair so well and deliver page after page of incredible, gorgeous fashion imagery that guarantees to get the creative juices flowing. My absolute favourites are books by Peter Lindbergh, Richard Avedon and Herb Ritts. And let's not forget the impact fashion has on hair. *Giorgio Armani* by Germano Celant and – obviously – Giorgio Armani (Guggenheim Museum Publications) is a favourite. The hair is everything you would expect from the fashion brand: sleek, androgynous and not to be messed with.

Magazines are an eternal source of inspiration: *Dazed, i-D, Vogue* (Paris, Italian, US and UK) and *Numéro* are must-have subscriptions.

GIRLS ON FILM

Movies are an endless source of both entertainment and inspiration for me. There are so many films that have stuck with me over the years because they deliver up incredible hair moments. The next time you have a quiet weekend stay in and binge-watch the following:

Empire Records (1995): Liv Tyler's hair sums up the look of the nineties.

Bonnie and Clyde (1967): Beret-wearing Faye Dunaway schools everyone in the perfect bob.

Pretty Woman (1990): Julia Roberts is one of the most beautiful women alive and even now, in her fifties, her hair is still out of this world. Her curls in Pretty Woman take some beating.

Sliding Doors (1998): If you're ever looking for an example of the perfect short crop it's Gwyneth's in *Sliding Doors*.

Wild Orchid (1989): Carré Otis's hair in this movie is wild and untamed and a great example of an eighties big hairstyle.

Dirty Dancing (1987): Jennifer Grey's uncontrollable curls in *Dirty Dancing* make her stand apart from everyone else in the movie – they all have groomed and restrained hair typical of the early sixties.

Tippi Hedren in any of her Hitchcock movies: Some of her films may have been in black-and-white but even then there's no denying Hedren's lustrous glossy blonde.

Clueless (1995): Most teens in the nineties wanted Cher's (Alicia Silverstone's) hair in this movie. But the inspo doesn't stop there; Tai's (Brittany Murphy's) bottled red colour was perfectly grungy and Dionne's (Stacey Dash's) braiding was another level.

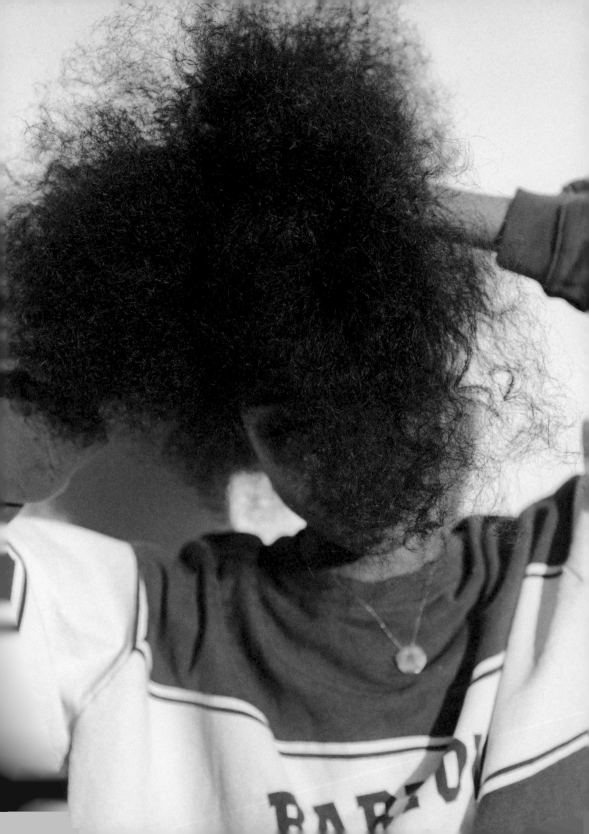

HAIR
TALK

A GLOSSARY

ANTIBOB

Where the traditional bob involves precision, the Antibob is a bit of an anarchist and based on a reverse-triangle shape that meets at the lowest point at the back of the head. The finished look is longer in the back and shorter in the front. The Antibob looks far more relaxed and effortless than a traditional bob and we're being asked to cut a lot more of them in the salon.

BAD BOB

A Bad Bob sounds rather sinister but it's really just an edgy bob cut with a Parisian feel and a hidden undercut around the back of the head. This is a style I created for Sienna Miller back in 2014 when she was working on a film and it looked awesome on her.

BALAYAGE

Balayage as a technique has actually been around for a few decades but really only became massively popular in the last six years or so. Most recognise balayage for its natural-looking multi-tonal look but few realise that it's painted on freehand – no cap or foils required. Because balayage is not one all-over colour, and instead a mix of complementary tones, it ages well and roots are less obvious as your hair grows.

BOB

A bob is a short, chin-length haircut that looks very classic and elegant when it's worn sleek and glossy. An iconic bob muse would be Faye Dunaway in *Bonnie and Clyde* but if you want more modern-day inspiration look no further than Bella Hadid who has recently been rocking the chicest bob.

CLIP-INS

Clip-in hair extensions enable you to go all out on volume with very little effort at all. A full set can come in a number of pieces (ours are made up of ten) and in a variety of shades. Again, clip-in extensions can be found in both synthetic hair and real human hair; the benefits of using real hair are that you can have it coloured to match your own shade exactly. They are super-easy to instal too: just divide your own hair into sections and clip the hairpieces against your scalp.

CURLING TONG / CURLING WAND

Most women are loosely aware of what curling tongs and curling wands are but they don't necessarily know the distinction between the two and which one they should be using. Both are designed to do one thing: to create a curl or a wave in hair. A curling tong comes with a clamp to hold the hair tightly against the barrel so that it absorbs a lot of heat, while a curling wand doesn't have a clamp and relies on you wrapping the hair around its barrel and holding it in place while it 'cooks'. A tong is best for anyone who has stubborn hair that's reluctant to curl – or when it does curl it easily drops out – whereas a wand is great for anyone who has chemically processed hair that curls very easily.

DETANGLERS

Detanglers are used in conditioners for obvious reasons. The most common ones are cetrimonium chloride and cetrimonium methosulfate. Brilliant for coarse and curly hair.

FATTY ALCOHOLS

Fatty alcohols often appear on conditioner labels as cetyl alcohol, stearyl alcohol or cetearyl alcohol, which, despite being alcohols, actually moisturise your hair.

FLAVE

The Flave is a flat wave and something I came up with while working on a London Fashion Week show for Jonathan Saunders. It involves using a straightening iron, instead of a curling tong, to make a wave by feeding the hair in a zigzag motion through the straighteners. This technique creates a very cool, very graphic shape in the hair.

HIGHLIGHTS

Highlights have been around for years and years and they're going nowhere soon. Highlights allow your colourist to bring areas of light to your hair with either dye or bleach. The highlights of the nineties had a very bad reputation for making hair obviously stripy, but now highlighting is far subtler and the parts that have been lightened seamlessly blend in with the rest of your hair.

INVISIBLE LAYERS
Invisible layers work in the opposite fashion to traditional layers. Whereas traditional layers are cut into the top sections of your hair and are visible to the eye, invisible layers are cut into the *underneath* of your hair where they are less obvious but do a brilliant job of removing some weight and encouraging natural movement.

THE MIDDY
A mid-length cut that stops just below your shoulders. The Middy has a weight to it – it still feels as though you have long hair and it's just about long enough that you can still tie it up should you want to. The length is so important – if it was to stop at the shoulders it could feel a little *Stepford*, but coming in just a little bit longer still keeps the look cool and chic. US beauty entrepreneur Emily Weiss really pulls this length off.

OMBRE
Ombre is sometimes confused with balayage but they are both very different hair-colouring techniques. Ombre hair is hair with dark roots that lighten progressively as the colour works its way down the hair until it meets lighter ends. It's essentially a graduating style of colour from dark to light, roots to tips. This doesn't necessarily always translate into natural-looking colours and it is very popular to take colour such as blue, pink or grey through the hair towards the ends.

PARABENS
Parabens are a group of chemicals that have been used for decades to prevent harmful bacteria from forming and preserve the shelf life of your products. They are a controversial ingredient that has received a lot of negative (much of it inaccurate) press over the years. Despite being demonised, parabens are deemed safe to use in small quantities in beauty products.

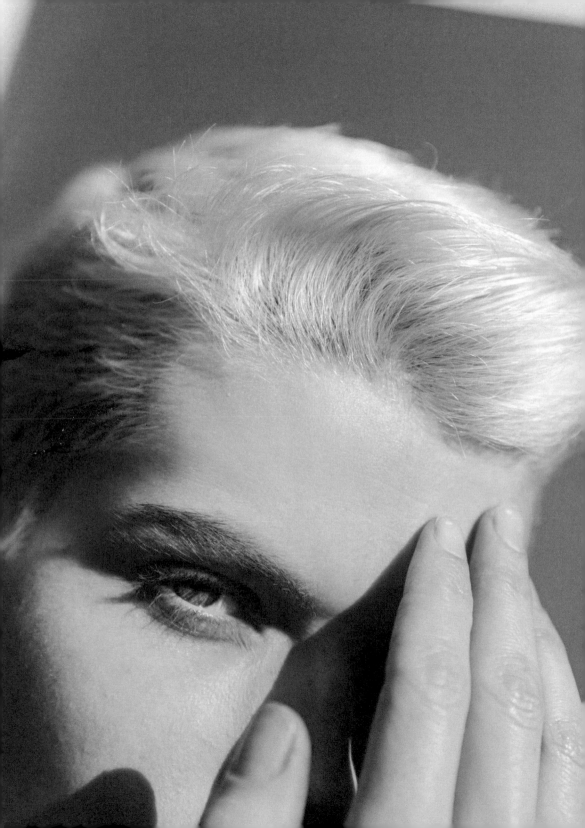

PERM

You're familiar with perming as a concept but the treatment itself is a far cry from what it used to be back in the eighties. The solutions are much the same – though they tend to be less damaging – but the technique is something entirely new. Gone is the one-size-fits-all poodle perm and in its place is something much more customisable. We sometimes set hair around foam pads to create a soft 'undone' wave and we sometimes do away with the pads and rollers altogether and just braid hair in perming solution to create a barely perceptible wave but masses of volume.

PERMANENT BLOW DRY

Hershesons was the first salon in the UK to put the Permanent Blow Dry on its menu and it is still on there today. The treatment involves pasting hair in a keratin concoction that relaxes curls and waves and reduces frizz. Despite being called 'permanent' the results will actually last around three to four months – but that's up to four months of smooth, easy-to-style and quick-to-blow-dry hair.

PERMANENT HAIR COLOUR

Unlike semis, permanent hair dyes need mixing up and contain an oxidiser (such as hydrogen peroxide) and ammonia plus, of course, the pigment for your new hair colour. They can result in greater damage than a semi but the colour lasts much longer so you have to get your hair done less frequently.

PLOPPING

This clever air-drying technique allows you to create soft, touchable and defined curls without any heat. It's really easy too; apply some styling cream to your freshly washed hair, lay a microfibre towel down on a table in front of you, bend your head upside down to 'plop' your hair into the centre of the towel, and fold the sides up to secure into the style of a turban. Go about your business while your hair dries and when you let it down you'll have perfect curls.

PRE-POO

This is a brilliant cleansing technique for anyone who has hair that doesn't agree with shampoo. Very curly, coily and Afro hair types can be very dry and brittle and shampooing can sometimes make it feel even drier and *more* brittle. To pre-poo involves applying a nourishing, oily and rich product – such as coconut oil – to the hair for a time to cleanse and hydrate. This can either be rinsed or shampooed out.

PROTEINS

Proteins – such as wheat proteins and soy amino acids – are used in conditioners and masks to give the hair strength.

RAZORING

In the simplest of terms, razoring means to cut hair with a razor rather than a pair of scissors. One way is not necessarily better than the other as they offer different benefits. Using a razor can give you soft and buttery ends while scissors tend to give you a more definite, sharper cut. Both have their place. I recently used a razor to cut Victoria Beckham's hair to her shoulders and it created the softest, most beautiful ends.

SALICYLIC ACID

Salicylic acid is a beta hydroxyl acid (or BHA) and it's used a lot in skincare products to keep pores clear of bacteria and treat acne. It works just as well on the scalp and that's why you'll find it in a lot of shampoos that have been formulated for flaky and easily irritated scalps.

SEMI-PERMANENT HAIR COLOUR

A semi-permanent hair colour delivers a natural-looking shade that lasts around six weeks before fading out. It doesn't contain any bleach, which makes it gentler on your hair but as the colour doesn't last too long you may find yourself having to get your hair done more often, which of course may result in some damage. The important thing to remember about a semi is that despite the name the colour will never actually fully leave your hair, it will just fade.

SHAG CUT

A shag is another one of those Seventies styles that have found a new lease of life in today's hairdressing. It's a short-ish cut with some thoughtfully placed layers that actually look randomly placed. The low maintenance look of a shag makes it look very cool. For shag inspiration look to fashion models Freja Beha Erichsen and Edie Campbell.

SILICONES

Silicones or siloxanes seal the hair's cuticle and make it shine. They have had a lot of bad things said about them over the years, primarily because they can't be rinsed away and need to be removed with shampoo so they can build up on the hair over time. This isn't necessarily a bad thing and you may have no problems at all with silicones, but they can feel heavy on very fine hair.

SODIUM CHLORIDE

Sodium chloride, essentially salt, is found in some shampoos. It roughs the cuticle up a little and so can make fine, flat hair look fuller. If your hair is very coarse you may not want to use a shampoo containing it.

SULPHATES

Common sulphates (often shown as sodium laureth sulfate, ammonium lauryl sulfate, sodium trideceth sulfate and cocamidopropyl betaine) are the main cleansing ingredient in shampoo and they're the ingredient that creates a lather.

TINT

A classic tint is an all-over permanent colour that is typically used to cover grey hair (it covers around 90 per cent of grey hair). Sometimes a tint may be used just at the roots if you're using highlights elsewhere, just to give the illusion of a darker root area.

TONER

Bleaching and colouring can make blondes appear brassy and yellow after a time. It's not a good look on anyone. A toner is a brilliant product because it deposits a touch of colour in a shade opposite yellow on the colour wheel (which happens to be blue and purple) that neutralises the brassiness without actually lifting the colour any lighter. It's clever stuff.

UNDERCUT
An undercut is a look that has been around since at least as early as the twenties but up until the last decade it was really only ever seen on men. It's a cut that combines both long hair (or longish hair) and an area of hair that has been shaved very short against the scalp. Rihanna is the queen of the undercut and has been seen with a variety of them – against both long and short hair – over the last few years.

WAVY GRAVY
We introduced Wavy Gravy to our blow dry menu way back in 2002 and it is still as popular as ever. It's dishevelled and laid-back and peppered with an irregular gutsy wave throughout. These are impossibly cool waves, very noughties, very easy to do but they make a real rock 'n' roll statement.

WINGE
A winge is essentially a clip-in fringe and gets its name from a combination of 'wig' and 'fringe'. A winge comes pre-coloured and pre-styled and can be made from synthetic hair or human hair. A synthetic hair winge retains its style without any maintenance. A winge instantly updates your hairstyle, it's easy to clip into your own hair and the best bit is that it requires zero commitment on your part.

ACKNOWLEDGEMENTS

Thank you to my family – my glue. To my dad Daniel, my best friend, who I've always looked up to. To my mum Ruth, sister Lauren and amazing wife Vicky. And my new reason for being, Marni my daughter. You're all so incredibly supportive of everything I do and you keep me in line, thank you.

I would also like to say a special thank you to Julietta Dexter, Jo Jones and Jess Wilcox at The Communications Store as well as Tania Bard for telling the world about Hershesons. To Christopher Miles and the team at Art and Commerce, Guido Palau, Kim Sion and Julian Watson for helping me build and manage my career so far. To John Frieda brands for having me as their Creative Director and to L'Oréal Professionnel for supporting our salons.

To my amazing assistants past and present – the best in the business; Syd Hayes, Jordan Garett, Carly Landau, Nick Latham, Gemma Moore, Roi Nadin, Sean Paul Nother, George Northwood and Ryan Wilkes. To Elliot Bute and Hannah Rooney for being a brilliant management team. To the entire Hershesons team for working beside me, for making me proud every day and for always going that extra mile.

To the editors who have helped shape my career – your support is worth more than you know – Lisa Armstrong, Nadine Baggott, Sophie Beresiner, Jessica Diner, Catherine Hancock, Sali Hughes, Sarah Jossel, Emma McCarthy, Joanna McGarry, Nicola Moulton, Sarah Mower, Alessandra Steinherr and Joely Walker.

I am beyond grateful to Victoria Beckham for generously writing the foreword – I'm so lucky to have your support, thank you.

This book is possible because of the tenacity and passion of editor Elen Jones at our publishers, Ebury and the amazing team there. The images in these pages were created in collaboration with the wonderful team of Tom Newton, Ninni Nummela, Claire Thomson Jonville, Julien Schmitt and Rosie Vogel Eades. And put into focus by Jesper Ander, Jelena Loutchko and Moses Voigt at Acne. THANK YOU ALL – I'm so proud of what we've done.

Most of all I want to thank two great women. Sali Hughes – for writing the most incredibly generous introduction – but also for helping me to plan and shape what this book was to become. Thanks to your generosity, patience and guidance we formulated the manifesto that formed the basis of this book and created the chapters within it. Thank you Sali, so so much – grateful doesn't begin to cover it. Finally thank you to Suzanne Scott for breathing life into our stories and helping them come alive in the pages of this book. I spent most of my school years skiving off and sweeping the floor of my dad's salon, so thank you for bringing our vision, passion and our world to life with your words. And for doing it in exactly the way I would have if I hadn't bunked off all those English lessons! You have brilliantly documented the many hours/days we spent putting together every element and detail of this book – and in a way that perfectly encapsulates who we are and what we do. Thank you, thank you – you're a great talent, a great person – and you have great hair!

PHOTOGRAPHY CREDITS

Photography © Tom Newton
Executive producers:
Etty Bellhouse and Araminta
Markes, Bellhouse Markes
Production assistants: Polly
Woollard and Sonny Casson
Art direction: Claire Thomson
Jonville
Hair stylist: Luke Hersheson
Hair stylist assistants: Jordan
Garrett and Nick Latham

Stylist: Julien Schmitt
Make-up artist: Ninni Numella,
Streeters
Make-up artist assistant: Shaunna
Taggart
Manicurist: Trish Lomax,
LGA Management
Casting: Rosie Vogel Eades
Lighting: Prolighting

10 9 8 7 6 5 4 3 2 1

Ebury Press, an imprint of Ebury Publishing,
20 Vauxhall Bridge Road,
London SW1V 2SA

Ebury Press is part of the Penguin Random House
group of companies whose addresses can be found
at global.penguinrandomhouse.com

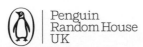

Copyright © Luke Hersheson 2018
Foreword © Victoria Beckham 2018
Introduction © Sali Hughes 2018

Luke Hersheson has asserted his right to be identified
as the author of this Work in accordance with the
Copyright, Designs and Patents Act 1988

First published in the United Kingdom by
Ebury Press in 2018

www.penguin.co.uk

A CIP catalogue record for this book is available from
the British Library

ISBN 9781785038785

Text by Suzanne Scott
Design by Acne
Art working and design by Louise Evans

Set in Optima Nova 9.3 pt & Harmonia Sans 6pt
Colour origination by Altaimage
Printed and bound in China by C&C Offset Printing Co., Ltd

Penguin Random House is committed to a sustainable
future for our business, our readers and our planet.
This book is made from Forest Stewardship Council®
certified paper.

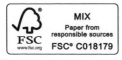